Major Incident Medical Management and Support

Major Incident Medical Management and Support

The Practical Approach at the Scene

FOURTH EDITION

Advanced Life Support Group

EDITED BY

Tony Gleeson

Kevin Mackway-Jones

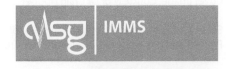

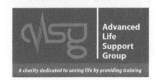

WILEY Blackwell

Registered Office(s)
John Wiley & Sons, Inc., 111 River Street, Hoboken, NJ 07030, USA
John Wiley & Sons Ltd, The Atrium, Southern Gate, Chichester, West Sussex, PO19 8SQ, UK

Editorial Office
9600 Garsington Road, Oxford, OX4 2DQ, UK

For details of our global editorial offices, customer services and more information about Wiley products visit us at www.wiley.com

Library of Congress Cataloging-in-Publication Data Applied for

Paperback ISBN: 9781119634669

Cover Design: Wiley
Cover Image: Courtesy of Dr Craig Hooper

Set in 10/12pt Myriad Light by Straive, Pondicherry, India
Printed and bound by CPI Group (UK) Ltd, Croydon, CR0 4YY

C9781119634669_230224

Contents

UK working group

Phil Bain	MBA, NEAS, NHS England (retired)
Tony Gleeson	B(Med)Sc MB BCh BAO AFRCSI DipIMC FRCEM FFSEM, Consultant in Emergency Medicine, Clinical Lead Emergency Planning, Salford Royal NHS Foundation Trust, MERIT Doctor North West Ambulance Service
Gary A. Hardacre	QAM, Scottish Ambulance Service (retired)
Zoë Hayman	MSc MCPara, Emergency Planning, Resilience and Response Officer, NHS England and NHS Improvement
Kevin Mackway-Jones	FRCP FRCS FRCEM, Consultant in Emergency Medicine, Manchester University NHS Foundation Trust, Director of Postgraduate Medicine, Manchester Metropolitan University
Jeff McClure	MCPara, Emergency Planning Officer, Northern Ireland Ambulance Service
Brodie Paterson	FRCS (A&E) FRCEM DIMC, Consultant in Emergency Medicine, NHS Tayside
Jonathan Taylor-Edmondson	MSc, Healthcare Emergency and Business Continuity Management, Trust Incident Manager, South Western Ambulance NHS Foundation Trust
Jamie Vassallo	PgCert DipIMC PhD, Emergency Medicine and Pre-Hospital Emergency Medicine Registrar, Post-Doctoral Research Fellow, Academic Department of Military Emergency Medicine
Darren Walter	FRCS FRCEM FIMC FAEMS, Senior Lecturer in Emergency Global Health, University of Manchester, Honorary Consultant in Emergency Medicine, Manchester University NHS Foundation Trust

International reference group

Australia

Andrew Pearce
BSc Hons BMBS FACEM PGCert Aeromed retrieval DRTM (RCSEd) GAICD, Emergency Medicine Consultant, Royal Adelaide Hospital and Director Clinical Services MedSTAR Emergency Medical Retrieval Service, South Australia

Egypt

Mohamed Rashad Abdelaziz
MBBS EMDM, Emergency/disaster Medicine Consultant, IFRC Medical delegate for MENA region

Atef Radwan
MD EMDM MSc JMHPE DHPE, Professor of Anesthesia, Consultant Intensivist, Head of Intensive Care Department, KASH, KSA

Japan

Naoto Morimura
MD PhD, Professor and Chair of Department of Emergency Medicine, Teikyo University School of Medicine, Visiting Professor of Department of Emergency Medicine, Yokohama City University Graduate School of Medicine

Taro Irisawa
MD PhD, Lecturer in Department of Traumatology and Acute Critical Medicine, Osaka University Graduate School of Medicine

Qatar

Walid Othman AbouGalala
MBBS JMC (EM) EMDM MSc, Consultant Emergency and Disaster Medicine, Executive Director Major Incident Planning, Hamad Medical Corporation

South Africa

Lee A. Wallis
MBChB MD FRCS FRCP FRCEM FIFEM, Head of Emergency Medicine, Western Cape Government. Professor and Head of Division of Emergency Medicine, University of Cape Town

Switzerland

Cedric Frioud
Paramedic with College of Higher VET Diploma, Educator with Advanced Federal Diploma of Higher Education, Lausanne Higher School for Paramedic, ES ASUR Le Mont-sur-Lausanne

Contributors to fourth edition

Phil Bain   MBA NEAS, NHS England (retired)

Ed Barnard   PhD FRCEM FIMC RCSEd, Consultant in Emergency and Pre-Hospital Emergency Medicine, UK Defence Medical Services, Senior Lecturer, Academic Department of Military Emergency Medicine, Royal Centre for Defence Medicine

Lieutenant Colonel Jon Barratt   MBBS FRCEM FIMC DMCC, Consultant in Emergency Medicine and Pre-Hospital Emergency Medicine, Defence Medical Services, University Hospitals of North Midlands and East Anglian Air Ambulance

Tony Gleeson   B(Med)Sc MB BCh BAO AFRCSI DipIMC FRCEM FFSEM, Consultant in Emergency Medicine, Clinical Lead Emergency Planning, Salford Royal NHS Foundation Trust, MERIT Doctor North West Ambulance Service

Gary A. Hardacre   QAM, Scottish Ambulance Service (retired)

Zoë Hayman   MSc MCPara, Emergency Planning, Resilience and Response Officer, NHS England and NHS Improvement

Kevin Mackway-Jones   FRCP FRCS FRCEM, Consultant in Emergency Medicine, Manchester University NHS Foundation Trust, Director of Postgraduate Medicine, Manchester Metropolitan University

Jeff McClure   MCPara, Emergency Planning Officer, Northern Ireland Ambulance Service

Andrew Pearce   BSc Hons BMBS FACEM PGCert Aeromed retrieval DRTM (RCSEd) GAICD, Emergency Medicine Consultant, Royal Adelaide Hospital and Director Clinical Services MedSTAR Emergency Medical Retrieval Service, South Australia

Jonathan Taylor-Edmondson   MSc, Healthcare Emergency and Business Continuity Management Trust Incident Manager, South Western Ambulance NHS Foundation Trust

Jamie Vassallo   PgCert DipIMC PhD, Emergency Medicine and Pre-Hospital Emergency Medicine Registrar, Post-Doctoral Research Fellow, Academic Department of Military Emergency Medicine

Contributors to previous editions

Contributors to third edition

Philip Bain	Emergency Planning and Resilience, North East Ambulance Service, UK
Jim Dickie	Emergency Planning and Resilience, Scottish Ambulance Service, UK
Peter Driscoll	Emergency Medicine, Manchester, UK
Peter-Marc Fortune	PICU, Manchester, UK
Tony Gleeson	Emergency Medicine, Manchester, UK
Gary Hardacre	Risk and Resilience, Scottish Ambulance Service, UK
Asiya Jelani	Ambulance Communications, Bolton, UK
Celia Kendrick	Emergency Nursing, Peterborough, UK
Caroline Leech	Emergency Medicine and Pre-hospital Care, Coventry, UK
Ian Norton	Director, Disaster Preparedness and Response National Critical Care and Trauma Response Centre (NCCTRC), Darwin, Australia
Darren Walter	Emergency Medicine, Manchester, UK

Editor

Kevin Mackway-Jones	FRCP FRCS FCEM, Professor of Emergency Medicine, Manchester, Honorary Civilian Consultant Adviser in Emergency Medicine, UK Defence Medical Services, Medical Director North West Ambulance Service, UK

Contributors to second edition

Simon Carley	Emergency Medicine, Manchester, UK
Denys Cato	Executive Officer, SWSAHS, Sydney, Australia
Timothy Hodgetts	Emergency Medicine, Defence Medical Services, UK
Paul Hustinx	Surgeon, Heerlen, Netherlands
Colville Laird	Immediate Care, Auchterarder, Scotland, UK
Kevin Mackway-Jones	Emergency Medicine, Manchester, UK
Per Örtenwall	Medical Director, Department of Emergency Planning and Education, Goteborg, Sweden
John Sammut	Emergency Medicine, Sydney, Australia

Contributors to first edition

Christopher Cahill	Emergency Medicine, Portsmouth, UK
Matthew Cooke	Emergency Medicine, Birmingham, UK
Patrick Corcoran	Fire and Rescue Service, Manchester, UK
Simon Davies	Emergency Nursing, Stoke on Trent, UK
Peter Driscoll	Emergency Medicine, Manchester, UK
Kenneth Dunn	Burns Surgery, Manchester, UK
Stephen Hawes	Emergency Medicine, Manchester, UK
Timothy Hodgetts	Emergency Medicine, Defence Medical Services, UK
Philip Jones	Ambulance Service, Manchester, UK

Colville Laird	Immediate Care, Auchterarder, Scotland, UK
Kevin Mackway-Jones	Emergency Medicine, Manchester, UK
Geoffrey Pike	Fire and Rescue Service, Manchester, UK
Stephen Southworth	Emergency Medicine, Manchester, UK
David Ward	Emergency Planning, North West Region, UK

Foreword to fourth edition

When the MIMMS course was developed in the early 1990s, the aim was to produce a course for healthcare professionals which used a simple structured system to respond to major incidents, to improve the quality of the health response at incidents and to integrate with the responses provided by other emergency services such as the fire and rescue service and the police. Indeed, concepts which were introduced in those early days have been adapted and used by the other services, METHANE as an acronym for declaring a major incident being a good example. Other countries were quick to recognise the importance of a structured health response at the scene and adapted the MIMMS generic concepts for use in their jurisdictions. Australia, Japan, Lithuania, the Republic of Ireland, Sweden and Switzerland have all adapted the principles and integrated them into their major incident responses. The MIMMs principles are in use in 15 countries and have been taught to over 22 150 candidates.

That structured system has remained an important part of major incident planning and response over the last 25 years, being used in many different responses including the 7/7 London Bombings (2005), the London Bridge Attack (2017) and the Manchester Arena Bombing (2017) to name but a few. Indeed, as I write we are still responding to the Covid-19 pandemic which, as a protracted major incident, uses many of the skills taught to candidates.

The principles have also been further developed and expanded by various organisations such as the Joint Emergency Services Interoperability Programme to produce the JESIP principles, joint decision model, logging, IIMARCH template and shared situational awareness amongst responding agencies and the National Ambulance Resilience Unit who developed command education and tabletop exercise writing and facilitation.

The fourth edition of the *Major Incident Medical Management and Support* (MIMMS) pre-hospital manual is still true to its origins, providing a succinct, easily readable text which conveys the key major incident messages for healthcare professionals. It provides an update on triage, a greater focus on the operational response and chapters on specialist areas such as planning for mass gatherings and firearms incidents. It is designed to provide the knowledge needed for a healthcare professional to understand and respond to an incident. The manual is the textbook for the MIMMS course.

I would commend the course and this manual to you.

Stephen Groves OBE
Director of EPRR
NHS England and NHS Improvement

Preface to fourth edition

'To fail to plan is to plan to fail'

Benjamin Franklin

When the authors of the first edition of this manual sat down 25 years ago, they had a vision to improve the knowledge and training of healthcare professionals in responding to major incidents in the pre-hospital environment.

They developed a manual and a course to train healthcare responders to respond to incidents in a professional way which would complement the other emergency services and work 'hand-in-glove' with them to improve the outcome for those casualties who were affected.

That their vision would provide a basis for a change that is still in use today, that has been used at some of the most difficult of emergency responses worldwide, is testament to the importance of that initial work they did to develop that MIMMS course.

The fourth edition of this manual seeks to expand on their seminal work and to bring it up to date. The manual can be used as a stand-alone text but is designed to complement a MIMMS course which has online learning components and face-to-face teaching and learning, to provide a comprehensive underpinning of the core knowledge needed to respond to an incident appropriately.

Tony Gleeson
Manchester 2022

Preface to first edition

'*It couldn't happen to us*' is not an acceptable excuse for being ill-prepared to deal with a major incident. A major incident may occur at anytime, anywhere.

Guidelines exist for the health services response to a major incident and these cover both the hospital and the scene. Each hospital must have its own Major Incident Plan and this should be regularly exercised. How well do we teach the principles of the major incident response to our medical and nursing staff? How much do we learn from our exercises? Are mistakes being repeated?

It is no longer acceptable to approach the scene of a major incident as an enthusiastic amateur. The transition from working in the emergency department to working at the scene does not simply involve putting on a reflective jacket and a pair of Wellington boots. The medical service must, like the police, fire and ambulance services, be skilled in command and communications, and have experience of the pre-hospital environment. This is in addition to coping with the enormous strain that mass casualties will place on the medical resources. To do this requires knowledge and training.

This manual, although a stand-alone text, has been prepared to accompany a course structured to teach the principles of management and support at a major incident to health service staff. This course will prepare both the Incident Officers, and other members of the scene medical response, for their duties in the event of a major incident.

T. J. Hodgetts
K. Mackway-Jones
Editorial Board
Manchester 1994

Acknowledgements

The development of this manual has not been possible without the dedication, enthusiasm and support of a large number of individuals who have given their time and effort to enable the continued development of MIMMS. We are ever grateful to the large number of instructors and candidates worldwide who have given feedback on how the course and manual content could be improved.

The authors continue to be grateful for the input of Mary Harrison and Helen Carruthers for their excellent line diagrams that accompany the text and would also like to acknowledge the input of Gareth Davis, Fiona Jewkes, Ian Maconochie, Graeme Spencer, Simon Swallow, Alison Walker and Ian Wilkinson to previous editions of the manual. The authors are grateful that their excellence provided a firm foundation to allow the text and diagrams to be developed further and expanded on, in this fourth edition.

The authors would like to especially thank Kirsten Baxter, Kate Denning and Julie Oliver of ALSG and the staff of Wiley-Blackwell for their on-going support and invaluable assistance in the production of this text.

Finally, we would like to express our deepest gratitude to Dr Kevin Mackway-Jones, who has decided to step down as chair of the working group. His contribution and dedication to the development of MIMMS from its inception to the current day has been remarkable and will continue to have influence in the years to come. We wish him the best of luck in his future endeavours.

Tony Gleeson
Chair, MIMMS Working Group

Contact details and further information

ALSG: www.alsg.org

For details on ALSG courses visit the website or contact:
Advanced Life Support Group
ALSG Centre for Training and Development
29–31 Ellesmere Street
Swinton, Manchester
M27 0LA
Tel: +44 (0)161 794 1999
Fax: +44 (0)161 794 9111
Email: enquiries@alsg.org

Clinicians practising in tropical and under-resourced healthcare systems are advised to read *International Maternal and Child Health Care – A Practical Manual for Hospitals Worldwide* (www.mcai.org.uk) which gives details of additional relevant illnesses not included in this text.

Updates

The material contained within this book is updated on a 5-yearly cycle. However, practice may change in the interim period. We will post any changes on the ALSG website, so we advise that you visit the website regularly to check for updates (www.alsg.org/uk/MIMMS). The website will provide you with a new page to download.

References

All references are available on the ALSG website www.alsg.org/uk/MIMMS.

Online feedback

It is important to ALSG that the contact with our providers continues after a course is completed. We now contact everyone 6 months after their course has taken place asking for online feedback on the course. This information is then used whenever the course is updated to ensure that the course provides optimum training to its participants.

How to use your textbook

The anytime, anywhere textbook

Wiley E-Text

Your textbook comes with free access to a **Wiley E-Text: Powered by VitalSource** version – a digital, interactive version of this textbook which you own as soon as you download it.

Your **Wiley E-Text** allows you to:

Search: Save time by finding terms and topics instantly in your book, your notes, even your whole library (once you've downloaded more textbooks)
Note and Highlight: Colour code, highlight and make digital notes right in the text so you can find them quickly and easily
Organise: Keep books, notes and class materials organised in folders inside the application
Share: Exchange notes and highlights with friends, classmates and study groups
Upgrade: Your textbook can be transferred when you need to change or upgrade computers
Link: Link directly from the page of your interactive textbook to all of the material contained on the companion website

The **Wiley E-Text** version will also allow you to copy and paste any photograph or illustration into assignments, presentations and your own notes.

To access your Wiley E-Text:

- Find the redemption code on the inside front cover of this book and carefully scratch away the top coating of the label.
- Go to https://online.vitalsource.co.uk and log in or create an account. Go to Redeem and enter your redemption code to add this book to your library.
- Or to download the Bookshelf application to your computer, tablet or mobile device go to www.vitalsource.com/software/bookshelf/downloads.
- Open the Bookshelf application on your computer and register for an account.
- Follow the registration process and enter your redemption code to download your digital book.
- If you have purchased this title as an e-book, access to your **Wiley E-Text** is available with proof of purchase within 90 days. Visit http://support.wiley.com to request a redemption code via the 'Live Chat' or 'Ask A Question' tabs.

The VitalSource Bookshelf can now be used to view your Wiley E-Text on iOS, Android and Kindle Fire!

- **For iOS:** Visit the app store to download the VitalSource Bookshelf: http://bit.ly/17ib3XS
- **For Android and Kindle Fire:** Visit the Google Play Market to download the VitalSource Bookshelf: http://bit.ly/BSAAGP

You can now sign in with the email address and password you used when you created your VitalSource Bookshelf Account.
Full E-Text support for mobile devices is available at: http://support.vitalsource.com

---

We hope you enjoy using your new textbook. Good luck with your studies!

PART I
Introduction

CHAPTER 1
Introduction

Learning outcomes

After reading this chapter you will be able to:
- Describe what defines a major incident
- Discuss the classifications of a major incident

1.1 What is a major incident?

In health service terms a major incident can be defined as any incident where the location, number, severity or type of live casualties requires extraordinary resources. The *number of casualties* alone does not determine a major incident for the health services. Thirty minor injuries that self-evacuate from the scene may be managed effectively by one hospital without the requirement for additional pre-hospital or hospital resources. The same number of *severely injured* casualties will almost certainly require extraordinary resources. Certain *medical resources* may be very scarce (for example, intensive care beds) or regionalised (for example, burns surgery), and small incidents with relatively few casualties can therefore require early involvement of regional or national resources. Where there are *large numbers of dead with few or no survivors*, there is often no major incident for the health services. An *incident in a remote or difficult* to access location may also demand greater resources to effect the rescue of casualties.

Factors that influence the declaration of a major incident for the health service

- Number of casualties
- Severity of injury
- Numbers of medical responders
- Access to medical resources
- Location (urban vs rural)

In a similar vein, *a major incident for one emergency service may not be a major incident for all other services*. Where fire or chemical spillage is the predominant issue, without risk to life, a major incident response will be required from the fire and rescue service without the same level of response from other services. Where public disorder is the predominant problem, the principal response will be from the police. The following examples illustrate this point:

On 2 September 1666 a fire started in a baker's shop on Pudding Lane; it lasted 4 days and left 80% of London's buildings in ruins. A disaster on such a scale is hard to imagine and would certainly overwhelm the resources of the modern fire and rescue service. In fact, only a handful of people died in this, the Great Fire of London.

Major Incident Medical Management and Support: The Practical Approach at the Scene, Fourth Edition.
Edited by Tony Gleeson and Kevin Mackway-Jones.
© 2023 John Wiley & Sons Ltd. Published 2023 by John Wiley & Sons Ltd.

On 27 March 1977 a KLM (Royal Dutch Airlines) Boeing 747 collided with a PanAM Boeing 747 aircraft during take-off in fog. All passengers and members of the crew died (total 583). This is the worst aviation disaster in history but had very little impact on the health response as all the casualties were dead.

In January 1975 a large petrol tanker hit the Tasman Bridge, a major transport structure linking the suburbs of Hobart, Tasmania. Thirteen people died, no one was left injured.

In April 1990 the passenger ferry *M/S Scandinavian Star* caught fire on the Swedish west coast. Most passengers were asleep and smoke inhalation caused the death of 158 people. The surviving passengers were mostly uninjured.

A health service major incident is influenced by:

1. Number of live casualties.
2. Severity of injuries.
3. Access to medical resources (ITU beds, burns beds).
4. Incident location (remote vs urban).

Local highlights: Major incident definitions

A major incident requiring extraordinary resources occurred three or four times per year in the UK (with a range from 0 to 11 incidents per annum) in the 30 years from 1966 to 1996. Although there is a particular emphasis on terrorist-related incidents in the west over the last two decades, it must be remembered that non-terrorist-related incidents continue to occur and are frequently associated with greater morbidity and mortality.

1.2 Classification of major incidents

It is convenient to classify major incidents in three ways:

1. Natural or man-made.
2. Simple or compound.
3. Compensated or uncompensated.

Natural incidents

A *natural* major incident is the result of a natural event such as an earthquake, flood, fire, volcano, tsunami, drought, famine or pestilence (Table 1.1). To some extent, the natural disaster will be self-propagating: following a flood or earthquake those left homeless and starving will be vulnerable to the diseases associated with squalor.

Table 1.1 Natural incidents (number of injured not accurately known)

Date	Type	Place	Estimated casualties
28 July 1976	Earthquake	T'angshan, China	655 000 dead
February 1983	Bushfires	Australia	76 dead, 1100 injured
19 September 1985	Earthquake	Mexico City, Mexico	40 000 dead
7 December 1988	Earthquake	Armenia	55 000 dead
17 January 1995	Earthquake	Kobe, Japan	6398 dead
27 June 1998	Earthquake	Adana-Ceyan, Turkey	145 dead, 1500 injured
26 December 2004	Tsunami	Indian Ocean	225 000 dead
12 May 2008	Earthquake	Great Sichuan, China	69 000 dead, 375 000 injured
12 January 2010	Earthquake	Haiti	220 000 dead, 300 000 injured
22 February 2011	Earthquake	Christchurch, New Zealand	185 dead, 2000 injured
11 March 2011	Earthquake and tsunami	Japan	21 000 dead, 5888 injured
27 December 2011	Floods	Philippines	Over 1500 dead, 1.6 million affected
29 October 2012	Hurricane Sandy	North America	Over 209 dead
7 November 2013	Typhoon Haiyan	Philippines and Vietnam	6150 dead
June–November 2014	Ebola epidemic	West Africa	Over 11 000 dead
25 April 2015	Earthquakes	Nepal	8857 dead, 21 952 injured
6 February 2016	Earthquake	Southern Taiwan	117 dead, 550 injured
September 2017	Hurricane Irma	Caribbean and Florida	134 dead
7 and 19 September 2016	Earthquakes	Mexico	350 dead
28 September 2018	Earthquake	Sulawesi, Indonesia	4340 dead, 10 700 injured
June 2019–October 2020	Floods	India	Over 4000 dead
4 April 2021	Tropical cyclone	East Timor, Indonesia and Australia	229 dead

Man-made incidents

The range of man-made incidents is huge, but certain patterns are clear. A major incident can occur whenever large numbers of people gather together to travel, to work or for leisure. In some circumstances, the incident will be the result of deliberate terrorist activity.

Transport incidents

These are the commonest type of man-made major incidents. All forms of bulk transport of people are associated with a serious list of incidents (Table 1.2). The worst ever road traffic accident occurred in the Salang tunnel in Afghanistan in 1982 when a petrol tanker exploded. Such was the degree of destruction that only an estimate could be made of the number of dead of between 1100 and 2700.

Table 1.2 Transport incidents

Date	Type	Place	Casualties
28 February 1975	London Underground crash	Moorgate, UK	43 dead, 74 injured
18 January 1977	Rail crash/bridge collapse	Granville, NSW, Australia	83 dead, 213 injured
2 June 1980	Rail crash	Storsund, Sweden	11 dead, 40 injured
22 August 1985	Aircraft fire	Manchester, UK	55 dead, 80 injured
6 March 1987	Ferry capsized	Zeebrugge, Belgium	137 dead, 402 injured
18 November 1987	Underground fire	King's Cross St Pancras Tube Station, London, UK	31 dead, 100 injured
22 December 1988	Aircraft bomb	Lockerbie, UK	270 dead
8 January 1989	Aircraft crash	Kegworth (M1), UK	47 dead, 79 injured
22 December 1989	Bus collision	Cowper, NSW, Australia	35 dead, 41 injured
27 December 1991	Aircraft crash	Gottröra, Sweden	34 dead, 115 injured
4 October 1992	Aircraft crash	Amsterdam, the Netherlands	34 dead, 7 injured
28 September 1994	Ferry *Estonia* sunk	The Baltic	860 dead, 137 injured
3 June 1998	Train accident	Eschede, Germany	101 dead, 88 injured
13 July 2005	Train accident	Sindh Province, Pakistan	127 dead, 800 injured
20 August 2008	Aircraft accident	Madrid Airport, Spain	154 dead, 18 injured
31 May 2009	Air France crash	North Atlantic Ocean	228 dead
13 January 2012	Costa Concordia grounding	Isola del Giglio, Italy	32 dead, 64 injured
8 March 2014	Malaysian Airlines flight 370 crash	Unknown (missing)	239 dead
28 December 2014	Indonesia Air Asia Flight 8501 crash	Java Sea	162 dead
29 October 2018	Lion Air flight 602 crash	Jakarta, Indonesia	189 dead
10 March 2019	Ethiopian Air flight 302 crash	Addis Ababa, Ethiopia	157 dead
5 May 2019	Aeroflot Air flight 1492 crash	Moscow, Russia	41 dead, 37 injured
27 March 2020	Subway train fire	New York, USA	1 dead, 16 injured
15 July 2020	Train crash	Czech Republic	1 dead, 35 injured
3 May 2021	Train accident/metro overpass collapse	Mexico City, Mexico	24 dead, 70 injured
7 June 2021	Train accident	Pakistan	50 dead, over 120 injured

Industrial incidents

The mining industry has been the site of a series of serious industrial major incidents (Table 1.3), but perhaps the most frightening incident to date has been the explosion of a nuclear reactor at Chernobyl on 5 April 1986, which left much of Europe contaminated with radioactive material. Around 40 000 inhabitants of Chernobyl were exposed to phenomenal levels of radiation for 6 days. The official toll of 31 dead, 1000 injured and 6000 losing their lives to cancer in the subsequent 70 years seem likely to be gross underestimates.

To some extent, the consequences of an industrial incident can be predicted. Local and national guidelines should exist for emergency planning at fixed chemical and nuclear installations and for the management of contaminated casualties.

Table 1.3 Industrial incidents			
Date	**Type**	**Place**	**Casualties**
14 October 1913	Explosion	Senghenydd coal mine, Wales	439 dead
21 October 1966	Land slide (slag heap)	Aberfan, Wales	147 dead
3 December 1982	Methyl isocyanate leak	Bhopal, India	8000 dead, 170 000 injured
6 July 1988	Explosion	Piper Alpha rig, North Sea	164 dead, 25 injured
2 August 1993	Chlorine gas leak	Stockholm, Sweden	0 dead, 33 injured
February 1996	Chemical truck fire	Sydney, NSW, Australia	0 dead, 60 injured
13 May 2000	Blast, fireworks factory	Enschedt, the Netherlands	17 dead, 947 injured
23 March 2005	Explosion, oil refinery	Texas City, USA	15 dead, 100 injured
11 July 2011	Gun powder explosion	Evangelos Florakis Naval Base, Cyprus	13 dead, 62 injured
17 April 2013	Fertiliser plant explosion	West, Texas, USA	14 dead, 160 injured
24 April 2013	Rana Plaza garment factory collapse	Bangladesh	1134 dead, 2500 injured
12 August 2015	Storage plant explosion	Port of Tianjin, China	173 dead
23 July 2018	Laos dam collapse	Champasak Province, Laos	40 dead, 98 missing, 6600 displaced
25 January 2019	Mining dam collapse	Chittagong, Bangladesh	233 dead

Mass gathering incidents

'Mass gathering' is difficult to properly define – but a working definition of the presence of a crowd in excess of 1000 people is in general use. Some of the worst tragedies have occurred at stadia around the world. Precipitating factors have included an overfilled stadium (Bolton, UK, 1946; Hillsborough, UK, 1989; Johannesburg, 2001), a crowd surge back into the stadium with a last-minute goal (Moscow, 1982), and a rush for shelter to escape a hailstorm (Kathmandu, 1988).

Events involving football fans prompted reviews of the safety of stadia and the statutory medical cover for such events. Reports have been published that give practical guidance for planning such events. More recently mass gathering public events such as pop concerts or religious festivals have led to incidents (Table 1.4).

Local highlights: Guidance for event planning

Table 1.4 Mass gathering event incidents

Date	Type	Place	Casualties
24 May 1964	Crush	Lima, Peru	318 dead, 500 injured
2 January 1971	Crush	Glasgow, UK	66 dead, 100 injured
3 December 1979	Crush	The Who concert, Cincinnati, USA	11 dead, 8 injured
20 October 1982	Crush	Moscow, Russia	340 dead, unknown injured
11 May 1985	Fire	Bradford, UK	55 dead, 200 injured
29 May 1985	Crush	Brussels, Belgium	41 dead, 437 injured
March 1988	Crush	Kathmandu, Nepal	100 dead, 300 injured
15 April 1989	Crush	Sheffield, UK	96 dead, 200 injured
13 January 1991	Riot	Orkney, South Africa	40 dead, 50 injured
12 October 1996	Seating collapse	Pink Floyd concert, London, UK	43 injured
16 October 1996	Crush	Mateo Flores, Guatemala	84 dead, 150 injured
30 June 2000	Overcrowding	Roskilde, Denmark	9 dead, 26 injured
11 April 2001	Collapse	Johannesburg, South Africa	43 dead, 155 injured
9 May 2001	Crush	Accra, Ghana	123 dead, unknown injured
29 March 2009	Crush	Abidjan, Ivory Coast	22 dead, 130 injured
24 July 2010	Crush	Love Parade, Duisburg, Germany	21 dead, 500 injured
13 August 2011	Stage collapse	Indiana State Fair, USA	7 dead, 58 injured
1 February 2012	Riot	Port Said Stadium, Egypt	79 dead, 500 injured
27 January 2012	Fire and crush	Kiss nightclub, Brazil	242 dead, 168 injured
11 May 2014	Stampede	Stade Tata Raphaël, Kinshasa, Democratic Republic of Congo	15 dead, 24 injured
21 November 2014	Stampede	Mbizo Stadium, Zimbabwe	11 dead, 40 injured
8 February 2015	Riot	30 June Stadium, Cairo, Egypt	20 dead
3 June 2017	Stampede	UEFA screening, Turin, Italy	1 dead, 1500 injured
22 August 2020	Stampede	Thomas Restobar nightclub, Lima, Peru	13 dead, 6 injured
30 April 2021	Stampede	Meron pilgrimage, Israel	45 dead

Terrorist incidents

The number of people killed or injured in the last two decades by terrorist bombs is so large that in some areas (for example, Iraq, Afghanistan) the toll is inestimable (Table 1.5). Secondary devices are frequently targeted at the emergency services, including the health service. Hospitals have also been the primary target. Any involvement of the health services that reduces the capability to manage the injured will result in a *compound* major incident.

Table 1.5 Terrorist incidents

Date	Place	Casualties
8 November 1987	Enniskillen, Northern Ireland	11 dead, 60 injured
26 February 1993	World Trade Centre, USA	5 dead, 1000 injured
20 April 1995	Oklahoma, USA	300 dead
30 July 1997	Jerusalem, Israel	15 dead, 170 injured
7 August 1998	American Embassy, Tanzania	5 dead, 72 injured
11 September 2001	World Trade Centre, USA	7700 dead, unknown injured
12 October 2002	Kuta, Bali	202 dead, 209 injured
11 March 2004	Madrid, Spain	191 dead, 1800 injured
7 July 2005	London, UK	52 dead, 700 injured
13 May 2008	Jaipur, India	63 dead, 216 injured
29 March 2010	Moscow metro system, Russia	40 dead, 100 injured
24 January 2011	Domodedovo Airport, Moscow, Russia	38 dead, 180 injured
22 July 2011	Oslo and Utoya Island attacks, Norway	77 dead, 319 injured
3–7 January 2015	Baga, Nigeria	Over 2000 dead
7 January 2015	Charlie Hebdo, Paris, France	12 dead, 11 injured
2 April 2015	Garissa University attack, Kenya	148 dead, 79 injured
31 October 2015	Metrojet, Russia, bombing	224 dead
13 November 2015	Paris attacks, France	35 dead, 340 injured
2 December 2015	San Bernardino, California, USA, shootings	16 dead, 24 injured
22 March 2016	Brussels Airport, Belgium, bombing	35 dead, 340 injured
1 June 2016	Dhaka, Bangladesh	29 dead, 50 injured
12 June 2016	Pulse nightclub, Florida, USA	50 dead, 53 injured
28 June 2016	Istanbul's Ataturk Airport attack, Turkey	42 dead, 230 injured
14 July 2016	Nice, France, truck attack	87 dead, 434 injured
19 December 2016	Berlin Christmas Market attack, Germany	12 dead, 49 injured
22 May 2017	Manchester Arena, Manchester, UK, bombing	22 dead, 500 injured
31 May 2017	Kabul, Afghanistan, car bombing	Over 150 dead, 413 injured
14 October 2017	Mogadishu, Somalia, suicide truck bomb	Over 500 dead, 316 injured
11–13 December 2018	Strasbourg, France, shooting/stabbing	6 dead, 12 injured
15 March 2019	Christchurch, New Zealand, shooting	51 dead, 49 injured
21 April 2019	Batticaola, Negombo and Colombo, Sri Lanka, bombing/shooting	258 dead, over 500 injured
3 August 2019	Texas, USA, shooting	23 dead, 23 injured
19 February 2020	Hanau, Germany, shooting	11 dead, 5 injured
2 November 2020	Vienna, Austria, shooting	5 dead, 23 injured

Simple and compound incidents

In a *simple* incident the infrastructure, that is the roads, the hospitals and the lines of communication, remain intact. When this infrastructure is damaged then the incident is said to be *compound*. The reasons for a compound major incident include:

- Damaged lines of transportation: roads disrupted by flood, earthquake or public disorder; poor weather preventing support helicopters from flying
- Damaged lines of communication: radio or cellular telephone 'black spot' at the scene; disruption of fixed communication lines
- Ineffective health services: services damaged by natural incident, as a result of terrorism or secondary contamination from casualties of a chemical incident

On 13 January 2010 a 7.0 magnitude earthquake hit Haiti. Significant damage to major infrastructure was sustained including: electricity, telecommunications, hospitals, transport (air, land and sea) and a large number of buildings, including the National Assembly, 60% of government buildings and the United Nations Stabilisation Mission buildings. The international aid effort was complicated significantly by the infrastructure damage. 3.5 million people were affected, 220 000 died and 300 000 were injured.

Compensated versus uncompensated incidents

A *compensated* incident is one in which the casualties can be dealt with by mobilising additional resources; that is, the 'load is less than the extraordinary capacity'.

In the Manchester bombing in 1996 the 212 injured were managed by paramedics and hospital mobile medical teams at the scene and transported to a number of hospitals for definitive treatment.

An *uncompensated* incident occurs when the additional medical resources mobilised by instituting major incident plans are still inadequate to cope with the number of casualties; that is, the 'load exceeds the extraordinary capacity'. This frequently occurs after *natural* major incidents such as an earthquake or flood (and these incidents are also often *compound*). *Man-made* incidents may occasionally be of such a magnitude that they exceed the capacity of the health resources.

The terms 'major incident', 'disaster' and 'catastrophe' are used interchangeably by some agencies and the media. Using the terminology discussed here, a 'disaster' or 'catastrophe' is synonymous with an *uncompensated* major incident.

> **Key point**
>
> In an *uncompensated* incident, the load of live casualties is greater than the surge capacity of the system.

Incidents involving children

Most major incidents involve a proportion of children and some predominantly involve children (Table 1.6). It is critical that major incident plans make appropriate provision for the effective triage, treatment and distribution of injured children to appropriate facilities. Preparation should ensure availability of an adequate and age-appropriate range of medical equipment/supplies to manage incidents involving children.

Table 1.6 Incidents involving children

Date	Place	Casualties
25 January 1990	Avianca plane, USA	73 dead, 159 injured
13 March 1996	Dunblane, Scotland, UK	18 dead, 15 injured
24 March 1998	Jonesboro, USA	5 dead, 15 injured
30 October 1998	Dance hall, Sweden	60 dead, 170 injured
22 July 2011	Oslo and Utoya Island attacks, Norway	77 dead, 319 injured
14 December 2012	Sandy Hook Elementary School, Connecticut, USA	28 dead, 2 injured
22 May 2017	Manchester Arena, Manchester, UK, bombing	22 dead, 500 injured
20 March 2019	Crema, Italy, bus hijack and arson	0 dead, 12 injured

Incidents involving burns

Mass casualty burns incidents can prove a significant challenge in that most expertise in relation to management of burns, particularly in the long-term management, resides in specialist burns centres. Coupled with this, there is a very limited number of specialist burns critical care beds available. It is likely that in a large burns major incident, mutual aid would be required across international borders. Major incident plans should incorporate how to access specialist advice for the management of burns patients, as in a major incident there may be a need for treatment of these patients in non-specialist burns centres. Table 1.7 shows incidents involving mass casualty burns.

Table 1.7 Incidents involving mass casualty burns

Date	Place	Casualties
14 February 1981	Stardust nightclub fire, Dublin, Ireland	48 dead, 214 injured
11 September 2001	World Trade Centre, USA	7700 dead, unknown injured
12 October 2002	Bali bombings	204 dead, 209 injured
20 February 2003	Station nightclub fire, Rhode Island, USA	100 dead, 230 injured
1 January 2009	Santika club, Bangkok, Thailand	66 dead, 222 injured
14 June 2017	Grenfell Tower, West London, UK	72 dead, 70 injured
2020–2021	India, 24 hospital fires	93 dead, unknown injured

1.3 Summary

- A major incident has occurred for the health service when the location, number, severity or type of live casualties requires extraordinary resources
- Major incidents can be natural or man-made, simple or compound and compensated or uncompensated
- Most major incidents in developed countries are man-made, simple and compensated

CHAPTER 2
The structured approach to major incidents

Learning outcomes

After reading this chapter you will be able to:
- Describe how you can prepare for a major incident
- Discuss the structured approach to major incident scene management
- Describe the structured approach to medical support at the scene
- Discuss how recovery occurs after a major incident

2.1 Preparing for a major incident

There are three distinct aspects to emergency preparedness. These are:

1. Preparation.
2. Response.
3. Recovery.

While man-made major incidents (for example, transport and stadia incidents) may be reduced by legislation and vigilance, natural incidents can only be anticipated. There are three elements to the medical preparation for a major incident: planning, equipment and training.

Planning

Failing to plan for a major incident is a sure way to increase the chances of failing on the day one actually occurs. 'It will never happen to us' is not an acceptable excuse for the absence of adequate planning.

The following plans must either be written by the health services themselves or must have appropriate links or health service input:

- An ambulance service major incident plan
- Plans for each hospital that are likely to receive major incident casualties
- Plans for high-risk venues (for example, major sports stadia)
- A regional/state/national plan for the coordination of resources on a wider scale

Plans need to be exercised on a regular basis to ensure familiarity with service responders, to ensure any potential faults are identified and to enable a review of the plan so it can be updated accordingly.

Major Incident Medical Management and Support: The Practical Approach at the Scene, Fourth Edition.
Edited by Tony Gleeson and Kevin Mackway-Jones.
© 2023 John Wiley & Sons Ltd. Published 2023 by John Wiley & Sons Ltd.

Local highlights: Major incident plans

Equipment

Personal protective equipment is required for all health service staff at the scene. There are also tools that may assist the health service commanders. Medical equipment should be matched to the skills of the provider. Doctors and nurses should bring appropriate equipment to the scene and this should complement not duplicate ambulance service equipment. These issues are discussed in Chapters 7 and 8.

Training

There are two aspects to training: education and exercise. It is important that education precedes exercise to avoid the repeated fundamental errors that have been demonstrated on multiagency exercises.

Education

The principles of patient assessment and treatment are those taught on advanced life support courses. These skills will be essential to members of the medical team but must be applied appropriately to the pre-hospital setting.

Major Incident Medical Management and Support (MIMMS) is a structured course for doctors, nurses and ambulance clinicians and managers that teaches a systematic approach. It has also been used to train emergency planning officers and some police, fire and military staff who will benefit from an understanding of this system.

MIMMS has been evaluated in a published attitudinal survey to detect any perceived change in ability to function at a major incident. One hundred per cent of respondents believed that MIMMS provided adequate training and all recorded a perceived ability to perform practical skills (radio procedure and triage) and function as a commander. The change in degree of confidence was most pronounced amongst the doctors and nurses.

Exercise

Exercises can take a number of forms. Exercising components of the response independently may facilitate a smoother full exercise:

- Table-top exercises to highlight communication chains and management structures
- Triage exercises with paper casualties or simulated live casualties
- Communication exercises to test staff activation cascades
- Practical exercises without casualties (PEWCs), walking the ground and responding to a developing virtual incident
- Multiagency exercises involving casualty handling, with or without processing casualties through the hospital, to test the hospital response

2.2 The structured response to a major incident

MIMMS provides a structured 'all-hazard' approach to the major incident scene response (major incident medical *management*) and to dealing with multiple casualties (major incident medical *support*), **irrespective of the nature of the incident**.

The 'all-hazard' structured response to a major incident can be adopted by the health service commanders at the scene and by all other members of the health services involved in the response. The approach involves seven key principles (Box 2.1). The principles have been shown to cross interservice, civilian–military and international boundaries.

Box 2.1 MIMMS management and support principles

Command
Safety
Communication
Assessment
Triage
Treatment
Transport

This is the 'ABC' of major incident medical response. The CSCA refers to the management of the major incident scene, whereas the TTT refers to the major incident scene medical support. Without a structured scene management system in place, the efficient medical support of casualties will be significantly impaired and hence the seven principles are hierarchical.

The CSCA key MIMMS management principles should be underpinned by the premise of emergency responders 'working together'. This can be better achieved if commanders:

- Co-locate as quickly as possible
- Communicate clearly using clear, plain language
- Coordinate by agreeing a lead agency and identifying priorities, resources and capabilities
- Understand risk by jointly sharing information on the likelihood and potential of hazards and threats and the agreement of control measures
- Have a shared situational awareness

Command

Each emergency service at the scene has a commander. 'Command' runs up and down (vertically) in each service. Overall responsibility will be taken by one service at the scene and this service is said to have control. 'Control' therefore runs across (horizontally) the services.

Ambulance commanders must ensure that they have command and control of the incident and this is achieved through the implementation of a command structure. The command structure of the health service is described in Chapter 3. The command structure and roles of the police, fire and support services are described in Chapters 4 and 5.

Control at the scene is facilitated by the use of cordons, which identify tiers of command at the scene. These tiers (referred to as Operational (Bronze), Tactical (Silver) and Strategic (Gold)) are described in Chapter 10.

Safety

The code of safety is remembered as the '1-2-3 of safety' (Box 2.2) and should be considered in that order.

Box 2.2 The 1-2-3 of safety

1. Self.
2. Scene.
3. Survivors.

Ambulance commanders must ensure the safety of all health responders, patients and members of the public. This is achieved through risk assessment and the identification and use of control measures.

Personal safety is paramount and is achieved by wearing the appropriate personal protective equipment (see Chapter 7). Where a hazard exists and either the training or the protective equipment of health service personnel is inadequate, then they should 'get out, stay out and call out'.

Safety of the scene is achieved by effective control of the cordons. The aim is to prevent those arriving to assist at the incident (or the media and public who will want to observe) from becoming part of the incident. Safety is discussed in more detail in Chapter 12.

Communication

Poor communication is the commonest failing at the scene of a major incident. Effective communication between the incident commanders must be established early and arrangements should be made for regular liaison in order to develop joint situational awareness. Radios are a common tool and staff who do not use them regularly must become familiar with radio procedure prior to the incident. Communications are dealt with in Chapter 13 and Appendix D.

Key point

The commonest failing of major incident management is poor communications.

Declaring a major incident

Each emergency service and every hospital that is capable of receiving emergency admissions will have a major incident plan that allows the rapid mobilisation of additional resources. The problem is often not the execution of the plan but rather a reluctance to institute it. This may occur for reasons of professional pride, for fear of criticism of over-reacting or out of ignorance. None of these is acceptable. If in any doubt, a major incident should be declared.

Confusion may arise at a hospital unless there is a clear message from the scene that a major incident has been declared and the hospital major incident plan is to be put into action. For this reason, it is important that the notifying messages to the hospital are standardised (Box 2.3).

Box 2.3 Major incident messages

1. ***Major incident – standby***

   The term used by an appointed member of staff to prefix messages indicating that an incident with the potential to generate a large number of casualties has or may have occurred.

   As the ambulance service is a gatekeeper to information, this message alerts wider healthcare that a major incident may need to be declared. It is therefore critical that this message is passed to hospitals that may have a role in any incident at the earliest opportunity.

   Major incident standby is likely to involve the participating NHS organisations in making preparatory arrangements appropriate to the incident.

2. ***Major incident declared – activate plan or confirmed***

   The term used by an appointed member of staff to prefix a message to confirm that a major incident has occurred, indicating that the plan should be implemented and a full predetermined attendance/response is required.
   This alerts wider healthcare organisations that they need to activate their plan and mobilise additional resources.

   Either of these orders can be rescinded at any time by the order:

3. ***Major incident – cancel***

   The term used to indicate that the state of 'standby' or 'declaration' is cancelled and actions should be stopped and normal operations resumed.

4. ***Major incident – stop***

   The term used by a commander to indicate that sufficient ambulance and/or medical resources are available at the scene and that no further assistance is required.

5. ***Major incident scene evacuation complete***

   The term used by a commander to indicate that the treatment and removal of casualties from the scene is complete.

   All receiving hospitals are alerted as soon as all live casualties have been removed from the site. Where possible, the Ambulance Commander will make it clear whether any casualties are still en route.

6. ***Major incident – stand down***

   The term used by a commander to indicate the conclusion of all ambulance service activity in connection with a declared major incident and a return to normal modes of operation.

   While ambulance services will notify the receiving hospital(s) that the scene is clear of live casualties, it is the responsibility of each NHS organisation to assess when it is appropriate for them to stand down their own response.

Other incidents categories

Globally there is recognition that some incident situations do not fully meet the criteria of the definition of a major incident and therefore do not constitute a formal declaration by the responding services. However, some incidents may still have an impact on the healthcare organisation in an adverse way unless a response plan is implemented. Examples of such incident categories include:

- **Significant incident –** any incident that, from initial intelligence, may require an attendance of a number of resources, a dedicated command focus or a specialist, dedicated or protracted response.
- **Critical incident – business continuity (internal incident only) –** any localised incident where the level of disruption results in the organisation temporarily or permanently losing its ability to deliver critical services, where patients may have been harmed or where the environment is not safe and requires special measures and support from other agencies to restore normal operating functions. Each will impact upon service delivery within the healthcare organisation and may undermine public confidence and require contingency plans to be implemented.

Additional measures and arrangements are put in place to effectively manage a response and maintain business across all healthcare service lines. A critical incident may be declared alongside a major incident if the definition is met and in order to protect operational service delivery of the healthcare organisation.

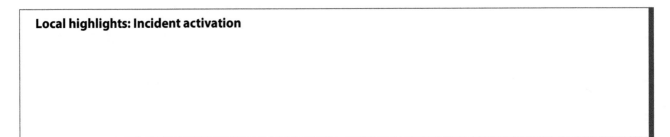

Local highlights: Incident activation

In some instances, casualties may arrive at the hospital before a clear message has been passed from the scene. In such cases the hospital should activate its own plan internally. For instance, in the Manchester bombing in 1996 only eight of 212 casualties arrived at hospital by ambulance and the decision to implement the major incident plan was made by the emergency departments.

Assessment

A rapid assessment of the scene is essential. Using information, intelligence, risk assessments and available policies and procedures, commanders must make a full assessment of the incident which is used to determine the initial health service response to the scene. From this assessment, commanders will develop the strategy and tactics for dealing with the incident. During the assessment phase commanders will identify the level and types of resources required to manage the incident.

The quality of the first information that is passed from the scene will be important in determining the speed and adequacy of the subsequent response. The acronym METHANE is recommended as a reminder of the key information to be passed (Box 2.4).

Box 2.4 First key information

M	**Major incident**	Confirm call-sign. Advise major incident 'standby' or 'declared'
E	**Exact location**	Grid reference, road names, landmarks, What3words, etc.
T	**Type of incident**	Rail, chemical, road traffic collision, etc.
H	**Hazards**	Actual and potential
A	**Access/egress**	Safe direction to approach and depart
N	**Number of casualties**	An estimate in the first instance and then upgraded with their severity/type (using triage categories, e.g. P1/P2/P3)
E	**Emergency services**	Present and/or required (be specific with required numbers)

Continuing assessment can use the HANE acronym (the second half of the METHANE message in Box 2.4). By continually reassessing the hazards, access, number and nature of casualties and the emergency services available to treat them, the incident commanders will ensure that they have the right people, with the right skills and equipment, to treat the casualties at the scene and the right transport to move the casualties to the right hospital for further care. This is discussed in Chapter 14.

Triage

This is the cornerstone of the medical support of casualties and involves the sorting of casualties into priorities for treatment. The process is dynamic (priorities may alter after treatment or while waiting for treatment) and must be repeated at every stage of the evacuation chain to detect changes. During a CBRN or active shooter incident the triage process may have to be modified. A simple system for triage is described in Chapter 15.

Treatment

The aim of treatment at a major incident is to 'do the most for the most', that is to maximise the benefit that can be achieved. The actual treatment delivered will reflect the skills of the providers, the severity of the injuries and the time the patient spends on the scene. The nature of the environment and the casualty load may restrict a provider's ability to perform to best practice standards. Treatment is discussed in Chapter 16.

Transport

In a conventional major incident in a developed country, most casualties will be moved to hospital by emergency ambulance or will make their own way there. Other forms of transport can be used and it is the responsibility of the health service commanders to ensure that patients are transported in an appropriate vehicle with the necessary in-transit care. The aim of evacuation at a major incident is to get 'the *right patient* to the *right place* in the *right time*'. Transport is dealt with in detail in Chapter 17.

2.3 Recovering from a major incident

The pre-hospital phase of a typical major incident (one that is man-made, simple and compensated) will often only last several hours. The phrase 'casualty evacuation complete' may mark the end of the concentrated activity at the scene but the additional strain on an individual hospital will be felt for many days or even weeks in its effect on routine operating lists and outpatients. The rehabilitation of some patients can take years.

Most of the hospital staff and many of the emergency service personnel will never have experienced such an event and, understandably, some will show the signs of stress. This may be immediate and during the incident, but an acute stress response is common immediately afterwards. Much less common is an insidious syndrome of reliving the events with flashbacks and nightmares resulting in anxiety, sleeplessness and poor performance at work, known as the post-traumatic stress disorder (PTSD).

There is a requirement in the immediate period following the incident to begin a combined process of operational debriefing to learn the lessons to improve future practice and psychological support to provide the necessary emotional support (and, rarely, formal psychiatric treatment) for those coming to terms with the event. The psychological aspects of major incidents are discussed in Appendix A.

2.4 Summary

- A major incident has three phases: preparation, response and recovery
- Preparation involves planning, organisation of equipment and training
- An 'all-hazard' approach is required when planning for a major incident
- Each incident can be managed with the same structured response
- MIMMS provides a simple, structured and effective approach to training health service personnel

PART II
Organisation

CHAPTER 3
Health service structure and roles

Learning outcomes

After reading this chapter you will be able to:
- Describe how the health services are structured during a major incident
- Describe who is in command of the ambulance and medical services at the scene
- Discuss who is in control of the health service response
- Describe the responsibilities of the Ambulance Incident Commander
- Describe the responsibilities of the Medical Advisor
- Define how the health service response is organised
- Discuss the medical and nursing staff involved and their functions

3.1 Command and control

Command and control are cornerstones of the major incident response. An understanding of the health service command and control is important, so that correct communications and management occur at the scene. Remember that in the initial stages of an incident, an individual may take on more than just one role, to ensure that all roles are filled. The hierarchy 'collapses' in this case and then as personnel arrive, the roles are allocated such that the hierarchy 'expands'.

Command structure (Figure 3.1)

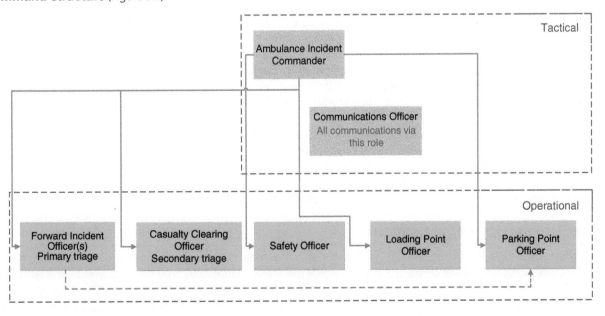

Figure 3.1 Command structure

Major Incident Medical Management and Support: The Practical Approach at the Scene, Fourth Edition.
Edited by Tony Gleeson and Kevin Mackway-Jones.
© 2023 John Wiley & Sons Ltd. Published 2023 by John Wiley & Sons Ltd.

1. The initial or interim Ambulance Incident Commander (AIC) role will be undertaken by the most appropriate member of the first ambulance to arrive on scene.
2. The other person on the vehicle will undertake the role of the Communications Officer.
3. These roles will be superseded by a senior officer and a control officer with the appropriate training and competencies.
4. The interim AIC and Communications Officer will be re-tasked into other officer positions or to respond to casualties as appropriate.
5. As further ambulances or officers arrive, the remaining positions will be filled as directed by the AIC.
6. The Forward Incident Officer(s) (FIO), dependant on the numbers of designated sectors, will be responsible for ensuring that primary triage is undertaken within the inner cordon.
7. The Casualty Clearing Officer (CCO) will be responsible for ensuring that secondary triage is undertaken within the Casualty Clearing Station and the casualty distribution to receiving hospitals based on their clinical needs.
8. The roles of Loading Point and Parking Point, although separate roles, may be undertaken by one person if the locations of the two positions are sufficiently close to manage both.
9. Although a dynamic risk assessment is undertaken by the AIC and any mitigating actions implemented to reduce any potential risks, the role of Safety Officer will be filled when resources allow and will continue monitoring the risks involved and staff welfare throughout the incident. All staff have a responsibility for safety (self, scene and survivors) and will be supported by the fire and rescue service with any specialist advice to ensure that the scene is sufficiently safe. It is still however the responsibility of the AIC for the overall safety of all health service personnel.

3.2 Ambulance services organisation

The ambulance service will provide the mainstay of the health response at the scene. Ambulance personnel are, on the whole, trained to work singly or in pairs to give care to a single casualty. Each unit operates independently and is tasked by an ambulance communications centre. In day-to-day operations, each unit acts alone without the supervision of an ambulance officer. If working in pairs then one member of the team leads the provision of care and the other assists in care and drives the vehicle. These roles will be referred to as attendant and assistant, respectively, throughout the rest of the text.

Ambulances services use a variety of vehicles on a day-to-day basis including emergency ambulances, rapid response cars, motorbikes and helicopters. They may also have major incident support units/mass casualty equipment vehicles and non-emergency vehicles that can be quickly deployed to an incident.

Ambulance service specialist teams

Some ambulance services have specialist teams that may be deployed according to a 'predetermined attendance' (PDA) procedure. This allows a number of highly equipped vehicles and trained personnel to be dispatched to specific types of incident based on hazard and risk assessments. These hazard and risk assessments will be reviewed and exercised on a regular basis. An example of this would be the response to airport, rail or hazardous materials incidents. It is also recognised that having a predetermined attendance to a major incident standby or declared major incident may be helpful in providing the initial number of resources to the incident scene in a timely fashion.

In the UK, the Hazardous Area Response Team (HART) is a specialist team trained in major incident response with the capability to operate in hazardous environments. Specific skills such as urban search and rescue (USAR), support to offshore incidents and support to police firearms teams may feature as part of their role. Special Operations Response Teams (SORTs) are specialist teams trained in major incident response, including the decontamination of casualties. In other countries, the fire service personnel have extended paramedic roles and in these cases the HART may come from within the fire service.

3.3 Medical services organisation

Increasingly, medical staff (doctors and nurses) responding in an official capacity to the scene of a major incident will come from a pre-hospital background and will be trained in pre-hospital medical response. They may be employed by the ambulance service itself or come from a charity service (such as the local Helicopter Emergency Medical Service (HEMS)). They will not only be comfortable with treatment of casualties in a pre-hospital environment but will also be trained in the major incident response.

Acute hospital and primary care medical services are most often arranged around clinical teams and services. Each organisation will vary in the level of care that it will be able to provide in the event of a major incident. It is important that if specialist medical teams are required on scene, they are not taken from the receiving hospitals and they are supported by pre-hospital colleagues whilst on scene.

In some areas, there may be organisations that are trained and experienced in providing medical care for emergencies in the pre-hospital environment. If available, their expertise should be incorporated into the planned attendance at any major incident.

Planning for a major incident is a vital part of overall organisational preparedness. Key elements of planning include the setting up of command and control structures within hospital services. This is dealt with in detail in *Major Incident Medical Management and Support: the practical approach in the hospital* (Wiley, 2019).

3.4 Command and control of the health service response

The health services response at the scene is led by the Tactical (Silver) AIC and the Medical Advisor. The designated individual in overall command of the health response will vary from jurisdiction to jurisdiction. These two officers liaise closely with each other and with the commanders from the fire and police services. The particular titles of these commanders will vary from country to country.

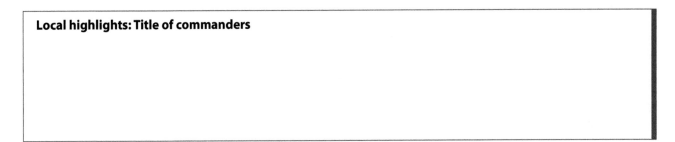

Local highlights: Title of commanders

Each commander wears a distinctive, chequered tabard inscribed front and back with their appointment, for example 'Police Commander'.

The AIC and Medical Advisor have distinct roles but must work closely together as a command team. This avoids duplicated or contradictory orders, reduces troublesome radio communications and allows difficult decisions to be shared.

In the UK, the AIC is *in control* of the response of the health services. Whereas in New South Wales, Australia, the state disaster plan clearly identifies that the Medical Advisor has control of the health service response.

3.5 Ambulance services at a major incident

Action of the first crew on the scene

The actions of the first ambulance crew at the scene of a major incident are critical in determining the speed of mobilisation of the health services and in ensuring that hospitals are given the maximum time to prepare to receive multiple casualties. Any delay in declaring a major incident by the initial ambulance service response may have a detrimental effect on the deployment of appropriate resources, the preparedness of the wider health services and in the health outcomes of the casualties.

Usually, if the initial response is a double-crewed vehicle, the ambulance attendant (the more medically qualified of the pair) will assume the role of initial Operational Ambulance Incident Commander and the assistant will remain with the vehicle to maintain communications with Ambulance Control (acting as the Communications Officer). The role of the initial AIC will be handed over to a more senior ambulance officer on their arrival.

Under normal circumstances, the first crew on the scene should not become involved in casualty treatment since this will stop them liaising with other services, assessing the scene as a whole and providing a continuous conduit of information as the incident develops. However, in some rural areas, where the travelling time to scene is greater, the crew may well have to initiate triage and treatment with support from the other agencies until other resources arrives.

The first substantial situation report (METHANE) will come from the first or initial AIC after a rapid assessment of the scene. The information that should be contained in this report is given in Box 3.1.

Box 3.1 Initial information to be passed from the scene of a major incident

M	**Major incident**	Confirm call-sign. Advise major incident 'standby' or 'declared'
E	**Exact location**	Grid reference, road names, landmarks, What3words, etc.
T	**Type of incident**	Rail, chemical, road traffic collision, etc.
H	**Hazards**	Actual and potential
A	**Access/egress**	Safe direction to approach/departure route to be agreed
N	**Number of casualties**	An estimate in the first instance and then upgraded with their severity/type (using triage categories, e.g. P1/P2/P3)
E	**Emergency services**	Present and/or required (be specific with required numbers)

The exact content of this initial report may vary. To ensure interoperability, local protocols should be followed.

Local highlights: Initial report

The first ambulance at the scene will become the Ambulance Forward Control Point and the Rendezvous Point for all health service resources arriving at the scene. All initial emergency services should co-locate at the same location in order to create the Forward Control Point (FCP). In the UK, the Ambulance Control Point (ACP) should be the only ambulance vehicle with its blue lights still operating. The use of this vehicle as the control point will be required until the ambulance service's designated control vehicle arrives.

The actions of the first ambulance crew on scene are summarised in Box 3.2. The attendant should identify a suitable location for the Casualty Clearing Station(s). At this early phase of the incident, this may involve no more than identifying an area or 'place of safety' where the walking wounded and uninjured survivors should gather and wait in the first instance.

Box 3.2 Actions of the first ambulance crew arriving on scene and the roles they should undertake

Communications officer (ambulance assistant)

- Park as near to the scene as safety permits
- Leave the blue lights on (indicating the vehicle is acting as the ACP)
- Confirm arrival at scene with Ambulance Control and provide initial, brief situation report
- Maintain communications with the attendant/AIC
- Stay with the vehicle until instructed by the AIC
- Leave the ignition keys in the vehicle

Ambulance incident commander (ambulance attendant)

- Undertake the role of the initial Operational Ambulance Incident Commander
- Wear appropriate AIC identification (for example, tabard)
- Commence a record of actions taken (incident log)
- Carry out a scene assessment (including a dynamic risk assessment)
- Give a 'critical message' to Ambulance Control (METHANE message)
- Declare a major incident/standby
- Identify the need for additional ambulance resources, medical teams or specialist/support equipment
- Identify key areas, for example, Ambulance Parking Point, Casualty Clearing Station, Loading Point, etc.
- Liaise with other emergency services at scene

Ambulance Control actions

On receipt of a METHANE message at Ambulance Control declaring a major incident or standby, the duty control manager should refer to standard operating procedures. There are two primary tasks: coordinating the response of ambulance service resources to the scene and ensuring that all necessary organisations and individuals have been informed. Examples of organisations that would need contacting include the police and fire services, local hospitals and local authority. Individuals that would need contacting include the call-in procedure for the ambulance personnel.

Ambulance service responsibilities at the scene

The responsibilities of the ambulance service at the scene are listed in Box 3.3. Their objectives are to provide the best possible care for the injured at the scene and to arrange rapid transport of the right casualty to the right hospital. Ambulance Control will have information regarding the capability and capacity at each local 'receiving' hospital and their ability to provide a medical team to the scene.

Box 3.3 Roles and responsibilities of the ambulance service at a major incident

- Establishing a forward control
- Saving life
- Preventing further injury
- Relieving suffering
- Liaising with other emergency services
- Determining the receiving hospitals – trauma centre vs trauma unit
- Mobilising necessary additional medical resources – Medical Advisor, Mobile Medical Team
- Providing communications for health service resources at the scene
- Determine a Casualty Clearing Station
- Determine the Ambulance Parking and Loading Points
- Determining the triage priorities for the treatment and evacuation of casualties
- Arranging means of transporting the injured
- Documenting the movement of casualties

3.6 Ambulance service key roles

To facilitate command at a major incident, a structured 'key role' approach is required. Roles are initially filled by crews as they arrive on the scene. Importantly, in the early stages an individual may take on more than one of the key roles to ensure that the key role actions are performed. Subsequently, as more individuals arrive on scene the roles can be allocated to individuals and handed on to more senior ambulance officers as they arrive. The use of key roles, rather than the specific appointment of officers to jobs, avoids the problems that arise when particular officers are unavailable or cannot reach the scene. The key roles are listed in Box 3.4 and their relationships to each other in Figure 3.2.

Box 3.4 Ambulance service key roles

- First crew on scene
- Ambulance Incident Commander
- Ambulance Tactical Advisor
- Ambulance Safety Officer
- Ambulance Communications Officer (on site)
- Forward Ambulance Incident Commander
- Casualty Clearing Officer
- Ambulance Loading Officer
- Ambulance Parking Officer
- Primary and Secondary Triage Officers
- Ambulance Equipment Officer

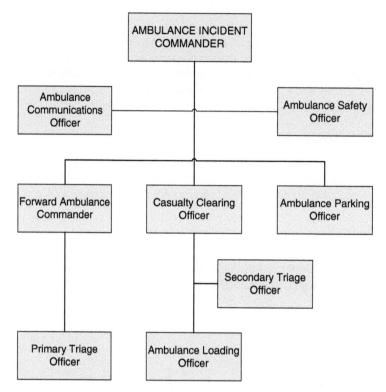

Figure 3.2 Ambulance service command structure

Ambulance Incident Commander

The Ambulance Incident Commander (AIC) is in command of ambulance resources at the scene, must not be involved directly with patient care and is identified by a distinctive coloured tabard which is clearly labelled. They can move anywhere about the scene but will usually stay close to the command vehicles and the other emergency service commanders to facilitate regular liaison. In the UK, the interoperability talk groups on the current digital radio facilitates the immediate contact of commanders without necessarily being beside each other. The following are the AIC's duties:

- Liaise with the Medical Advisor, Police Commander and Fire Commander
- Ensure the safety of ambulance and health service responders
- Delegate key tasks to other ambulance officers/personnel
- Ensure radio communications are provided to appropriate health personnel
- Carry out an assessment of the scene
- Determine where mobile medical teams are drawn from in liaison with the Medical Advisor (if on site)
- Determine which hospitals will receive casualties in liaison with the Medical Advisor
- Oversee triage and treatment provided by ambulance personnel
- Organise the most suitable transport for casualties
- Confirm access and egress routes for health service vehicles with the police
- Determine the need for support from voluntary agencies in an ambulance aid role and to oversee treatment provided by these personnel
- Arrange for replenishment of equipment
- Liaise with the police regarding media briefings

Local highlights: Ambulance service command structure

Ambulance Tactical Advisor

The Ambulance Tactical Advisor is a member of staff who has the relevant depth of knowledge regarding ambulance service and health service specialist and non-specialist capabilities, associated risks and the benefits of deploying and utilising such capabilities. The Tactical Advisor must have an in-depth knowledge of the response plan, and other relevant policies, doctrine and procedures.

Ambulance Safety Officer(s)

The AIC will delegate an officer to be responsible for the safety of **all health personnel** on site. Their duties include the following:

- Ensure that all health personnel are wearing suitable personal protective equipment
- Monitor staff for fatigue or stress and advise on the need to relieve staff
- Identify hazards, evaluate risks and ensure that appropriate control measures are undertaken
- Liaise with the other emergency services on safety matters and procedures
- Consider issues regarding contaminated casualties, staff, vehicles and equipment

---

Key point

Personnel who are not equipped with the correct personal protective equipment will be refused admission to the scene.

Ambulance Communications Officer

This officer provides and coordinates all on-site and off-site communications for appropriate ambulance and medical staff and communications between the ambulance service and other emergency services. The Ambulance Communications Officer is located at the Ambulance Control Point. Duties include the following:

- Provide a link between the site and main Ambulance Control
- Provide a link between the on-site Ambulance Command Vehicle and other emergency service incident control vehicles
- Provide a link between the site and the receiving hospitals
- Determine the most suitable communication mode for a particular message including radio, telephone landlines and cellular telephone
- Maintain a log of all transmissions from the health personnel at the site

Forward Ambulance Incident Commander(s)

This commander is responsible to the Tactical AIC for the management of ambulance resources in a specific sector/operational area. The Operational AIC works from the forward operational area/sector and is the eyes and ears of the Tactical AIC in that area. There may be a number of operational commanders depending on the size or type of incident. Duties include the following:

- Directing resources to ensure adequate primary triage
- Overseeing the treatment of trapped casualties
- Supervising the evacuation of patients to the Casualty Clearing Station (CCS)

Casualty Clearing Officer

This officer will confirm with the Operational AIC the site of the CCS. The following factors should be considered:

- The CCS should be a safe distance from all hazards
- The position should avoid long or difficult transport of patients from the incident site
- Natural shelter or buildings should be used where available
- There must be easy access for vehicles to load patients

The priority when setting up an initial CCS is to provide a treatment facility. This means identifying a piece of ground and opening treatment packs, boxes or rucksacks. There should be no delay in establishing this facility because of delays in erecting tents or any other temporary shelters.

The Casualty Clearing Officer will also:

- Establish and monitor secondary triage for casualties brought to the CCS, ensuring the triage cards are fully completed and stay with the patient
- Liaise with the Ambulance Loading Officer for transportation needs and priorities of evacuation and maintaining records of patient movements from the scene
- Brief and monitor medical staff working in the CCS
- Ensure there is adequate equipment within the CCS
- Keep the AIC informed about casualty numbers, severity and movements

Ambulance Loading Officer

This officer supervises the Ambulance Loading Point. Duties include the following:

- Liaison with the police to ensure that there is a protected route for ambulances to access the Loading Point
- Link with the Ambulance Parking Officer to call vehicles forward to the CCS as required
- In liaison with the Casualty Clearing Officer, decide on the most appropriate form of transport (including public transport, fixed wing aircraft, helicopter or boat)
- In conjunction with the Ambulance Equipment Officer, arrange the collection and return of all ambulance and medical equipment at the end of the incident

Ambulance Parking Officer

This officer will work from the Ambulance Parking Point. They will:

- Ensure the best utilisation of vehicle resources
- Maintain a log of staff and their vehicles attending the site (including the qualifications of attending ambulance staff)
- In conjunction with the AIC, send the appropriate ambulance personnel to the desired location

Local highlights: Ambulance service key roles

3.7 Medical services at a major incident

The medical services can support and enhance the ambulance service response as shown in Box 3.5.

Box 3.5 Medical aid to the ambulance service

- Support for secondary triage (triage sort)
- Perform advanced clinical interventions
- Perform emergency surgical procedures to facilitate extrication
- Treat and discharge casualties with minor injuries only at scene

3.8 Medical command appointments

The command appointments allocated to the medical services are shown in Figure 3.3. These are complementary to the ambulance service appointments. The responsibilities of the various appointees are described in this section.

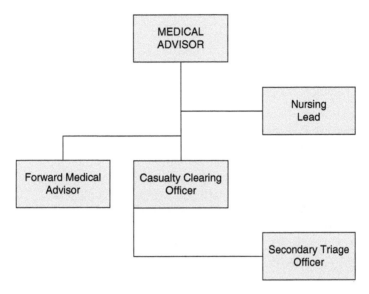

Figure 3.3 Medical service command structure

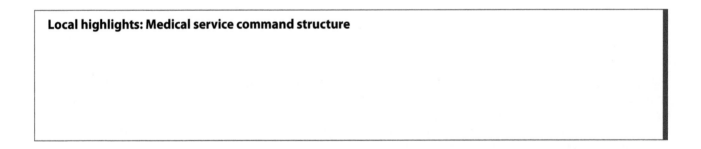

Local highlights: Medical service command structure

Medical Advisor

The Medical Advisor will usually take responsibility for organising clinical care at the scene or at a Tactical Coordination Centre but, like the AIC, must not be involved directly with clinical care as this would compromise the advisor role. Where required to attend the scene of the incident, the Medical Advisor should liaise with the AIC and receive a full briefing. The Medical Advisor can move about the scene but to be most effective should work closely with the AIC and other emergency service commanders. The Medical Advisor may be an advisory role only that carries no command authority, nevertheless their advice will directly influence the command decisions taken by the AIC, as in the UK.

The Medical Advisor should be identified by a clearly labelled tabard. Personal protective equipment for the Medical Advisor may be held by the ambulance service in their equipment vehicle or within a hospital major incident storeroom and may be issued in advance to individuals on a Medical Advisor's rota.

Local highlights: Command equipment provision

The following are the Medical Advisor's duties:

- Liaise with the AIC, Police Commander and Fire Commander
- Delegate key tasks to other clinical personnel
- Establish and maintain a flow of information to receiving hospitals
- Carry out a clinical assessment of the scene
- Establish specialist medical equipment needs and liaise with the AIC to ensure supply
- Determine whether there is the need for additional medical personnel at the scene
- Determine which hospitals will receive casualties in liaison with the AIC
- Ensure effective secondary triage is established
- Oversee the management of treatment provided by medical teams at the scene
- Liaise with the police and AICs regarding media briefings

The background of the individual acting as Medical Advisor is less important than the fact they have been adequately trained and have exercised in the role. The important competencies for a Medical Advisor are:

- Major incident management training and experience
- Pre-hospital training and experience
- An understanding of the logistics of the local ambulance service
- Local knowledge of hospital facilities and capabilities

All clinical staff arriving on scene should be briefed and tasked by the Medical Advisor. The Medical Advisor must ensure that clinicians understand and use the correct routes of communication. On completion of specific tasks, personnel should report to the Medical Advisor or a nominated representative for redeployment. A failure to ensure that this happens will allow other emergency service personnel to direct the clinical staff where they perceive the need. This will rapidly cause failure of medical command and ultimately be detrimental for casualties.

The Medical Advisor is also responsible for any doctors or nurses responding to the major incident in an unofficial capacity (for example, those who are acting in a good Samaritan way to the incident). It is important that the Medical Advisor ensures that he/she is happy that the individual is appropriately qualified, and appropriately briefed as above. Contact details of any good Samaritans responding should be kept for the subsequent incident inquiry and also to ensure these individuals get appropriate post-incident support.

Although the Medical Advisor has overall responsibility for the safety of clinical personnel, this will usually be delegated to the Ambulance Safety Officer. An initial assessment of the scene, made with the AIC, will help to determine the scale and nature of the clinical resources that are needed. Where resources allow it, the Medical Advisor may release clinicians to assist in primary triage. The Medical Advisor must ensure that effective secondary triage is performed at the CCS and repeated appropriately. By providing adequate personnel with the right skill mix, they will oversee the delivery of the best possible treatment for all casualties.

Forward Medical Advisor

Depending on appropriately trained resources, risk assessment and the agreement of the AIC, this role may or may not feature as part of the incident management structure. This doctor is the eyes and ears of the Medical Advisor within the forward operational area/sector. They should have no direct involvement in patient treatment, and act in an advisory role.

The principal task is the supervision of clinical and paramedical staff working in a forward area. Requests for a clinician or medical team to attend a casualty who is trapped must be directed through the Operational AIC to the Forward Doctor and by no other route. It follows that the Forward Doctor should work in close collaboration with the Operational AIC within each sector/operational area.

CCS Medical Lead Doctor(s)

The role would be a suitably trained doctor who takes responsibility for coordinating, supporting and advising paramedic and medical staff in the Casualty Clearing Station (CCS) to maximise the clinical care of all patients attending the CCS.

Key point

Ambulance Incident Commanders and Medical Advisors must never become involved with treating individual casualties.

3.9 Clinical staff at the scene

Hospital teams

Medical teams are often requested to attend the scene to assist the ambulance service. However, due to the geographical spread of trauma units, the provision of such teams may be limited. Medical teams coming from a non-receiving hospital may have very limited or no pre-hospital medical experience. It is often an ambulance service responsibility to arrange transport to the scene, which will be by marked emergency vehicle. If no ambulance is available, the police may be requested to assist with transport.

Once on scene, the team should have an allocated pre-hospital clinician to support them. The team leader of each medical team is responsible for the team's safety. This responsibility will have started in the hospital prior to leaving for the scene and will end only after each team member has been debriefed both operationally and emotionally. Only the team leader should accept tasks and team members should be tasked by their leader.

Hospital-based medical teams will usually deploy with no capability to sustain themselves in the field. They are reliant on the health service's command structure for transport, communications, food and water, shelter and any other personal needs. While this may cause few problems for incidents of short duration, natural incidents that require a protracted response with rest and rotation of staff in the field will unmask the lack of field-craft in such personnel. A degradation of clinical effectiveness is inevitable.

The medical team may be broken up and allocated a number of tasks or may be kept together and allocated to a treatment area. If personnel are deployed forward to the site of the incident, they will be under the immediate control of the Forward Medical Advisor; if they are working in the CCS, then the Casualty Clearing Officer will oversee them. Since all incidents are different, the exact nature of the team tasks and their relative priority will change. Tasks that may be undertaken, depending on the circumstances, include those shown in Box 3.6.

Box 3.6 Mobile medical team tasks

- Treatment of casualties at the site
- Secondary triage in the Casualty Clearing Station
- Treatment in the Casualty Clearing Station
- Assistance to a mobile surgical team if present
- Confirming death and labelling of the dead at the scene

The request for a mobile medical team will be a rare occurrence in most hospitals, and an action card is an effective prompt in this situation. This may include a reminder of who should be in the team, what immediate preparations are required, what equipment is needed (and where it can be found), how the team should move to the scene and what their initial actions are on arrival. An example of an action card listing the immediate actions of a mobile medical team is shown in Box 3.7.

Key point

It is an ambulance service responsibility to arrange transport to the scene for the mobile medical teams.

Box 3.7 Mobile medical team action card

Immediate actions

1. On being nominated as a member of the mobile medical team, proceed immediately to the emergency department.
2. Collect medical equipment and clothing from the major incident store. One nurse should obtain and sign for the major incident controlled drugs.
3. Once an ambulance arrives to transport the team to the scene, the team should load it with all the major incident equipment except that for the mobile surgical team.
4. Check that no special orders for equipment have been made by the Medical Advisor and then proceed to the incident site in the ambulance.
5. On arrival at the site, report to the Medical Advisor at the Ambulance Control Point for orders.
6. Under the direction of the Medical Advisor undertake all actions as required.

The medical personnel in these teams form a small but highly skilled part of the health service response. It is essential that their skills are used effectively and that they complement rather than challenge the role of ambulance personnel.

Clinicians deployed to treat patients at the scene must be properly equipped to work in the pre-hospital environment (both personally and medically) and must have the right clinical skills and experience for the role they have to fulfil. If these criteria are met, the extra skills available will benefit the casualties immensely. If they are ill equipped, inexperienced, inadequately skilled or undisciplined then they may pose a threat to the welfare of the casualties and other rescuers.

Local highlights: Mobile medical team capacity and provision

The need for a surgeon at the scene is rare, but occasions do occur (for example, when amputation or disarticulation is necessary to facilitate extrication). Surgical capability should only be summoned at the request of the AIC or Medical Advisor. A mobile surgical team, consisting of a capable senior surgeon, a similarly capable anaesthetist and appropriate scrub and anaesthetic nurse support, may be formed at a receiving hospital and dispatched via ambulance to the scene. This team will work under the close supervision of the Operational AIC (or Forward Doctor when present) and should return to the hospital with the patient after the surgical procedure is completed.

Local highlights: Mobile surgical team capacity and provision

---

Voluntary aid societies

Clinicians who are members of voluntary aid societies may be working at the scene either because they were already deployed (for example, at a mass gathering) or because they are mobilised to assist by the statutory ambulance service. These individuals will operate under the ambulance service's command structure.

Local highlights: Voluntary aid societies

Health workers involved incidentally

In most incidents there will be some health workers who become involved, either because they were survivors of the incident or because they were passing in the early stages. It is most unlikely that these staff will be equipped to provide anything more than basic first aid; furthermore, their lack of proper personal protective equipment means that they are at considerable extra personal risk. The emergency service and medical staff who have been mobilised to the scene should therefore take over as soon as possible. Health care staff who were involved in the incident should be treated like any other casualty, and those who have become incidentally involved should be given tasks away from the dangers of the scene itself.

3.10 Summary

- The Ambulance Incident Commanders and Medical Advisors are in charge of the health service response at the scene and must work closely together
- Ambulance personnel and medical teams will work within the key areas and will be under the command of the forward officers in those areas
- Clinical staff have skills that are complementary to the ambulance service
- Immediate care doctors and hospital-based teams must be properly equipped, trained, experienced and disciplined
- The exact nature and priority of tasks for a medical team will vary with each incident. In general, they will involve triage, treatment and packaging for transport
- Surgical input at the scene should be limited and should be task specific

CHAPTER 4
Emergency service organisation and roles

Learning outcomes

After reading this chapter you will be able to:
- Describe the role and organisation of the police service at a major incident
- Describe the role and organisation of the fire and rescue service at a major incident
- Describe the role and organisation of the maritime and coastguard services at a major incident

---

4.1 Organisation

It is essential that health service staff understand the organisation and roles of the other emergency services. As with the ambulance service, the police, fire and rescue service and maritime and coastguard services are hierarchical with clear command and control systems and rank structures.

4.2 Role of the police at a major incident

In many domains, the police service have overall responsibility to coordinate the multiagency actions at the scene of a major incident. When a hazard is present (such as fire or chemical spillage), the police will surrender initial control of the *immediate* scene area within the inner cordon (Operational (Bronze) area) to the fire and rescue service.

Police Control, in line with all other emergency controls, has a responsibility to inform other emergency services when the major incident plan is activated.

The initial responsibilities of the police are given in Box 4.1.

Box 4.1 Initial responsibilities of the police

- Command and control of the incident and establishing a Forward Control
- Commencing and maintaining an incident log
- Saving life in conjunction with other emergency services
- Preventing escalation of the incident
- Evacuating those still in danger
- Ensuring the activation of other emergency services
- Providing traffic management and identifying access and egress for emergency services
- Liaising with and facilitating other emergency services
- Maintaining records of the casualties and uninjured survivors
- Identifying the dead and liaising with the coronial/procurator fiscal services
- Maintaining public order
- Protecting property
- Criminal investigation and assisting with official enquiries
- Liaising with the media

Major Incident Medical Management and Support: The Practical Approach at the Scene, Fourth Edition.
Edited by Tony Gleeson and Kevin Mackway-Jones.
© 2023 John Wiley & Sons Ltd. Published 2023 by John Wiley & Sons Ltd.

Members of the public who are in imminent danger after the incident (for instance from fire, chemical exposure or radioactive contamination) must be evacuated to safety by the emergency services. Police officers will establish an outer cordon at a position that limits access by the general public but supports the access and egress of the emergency services responding. Once established, they will also record the names of emergency service workers requiring access.

Management of uninjured survivors

The police service may request that the local civil authority establish a Survivor Reception Centre at an appropriate location that will provide basic welfare needs. The local civil authority will provide food and refreshment at this location while health services need to provide clinical care.

Survivors are regarded as witnesses to what often becomes a criminal enquiry. At first it may only be appropriate to take names and addresses at the Survivor Reception Centre as individuals may be too distressed to provide a full statement. The requirements for a Survivor Reception Centre are listed in Box 4.2.

Box 4.2 Requirements for a Survivor Reception Centre

- Secure area away from the public and press
- Food
- Water
- Sanitation
- Dry clothing
- Documentation
- Social care
- Clinical care

Management of friends and relatives

Friends and relatives who were not involved in the incident may make their way to the scene. They should receive appropriate advice from the police and local authorities which may include casualty bureau contact numbers, helpline numbers, etc.

Management of the dead

In most countries, death can only be diagnosed by a trained clinician. Identification of the dead is a key role often overseen by the Police Commander.

When authority is granted to move a body, it is the responsibility of the police service to do this. It is the decision of the Coroner/fiscal agency as to whether a temporary mortuary should be established. The purpose of a temporary mortuary is for the forensic pathological examination and formal identification of the dead.

Traffic management

The maintenance of free traffic flow and the organisation of vehicle marshalling areas ensure the continued smooth running of the incident.

Law and order

The scene of a major incident is a potential scene of crime. Evidence must be protected for use in later criminal investigations.

Police aid to the health services

The police can assist the medical services at the scene of a major incident in the ways shown in Box 4.3.

Box 4.3 Police aid to the medical services

- Assist with the transport of medical personnel either directly or by providing an escort (local agreement)
- Maintain clear transport routes to ensure the uninhibited movement of ambulances
- Provide escorts for individual casualties to hospital (local agreement)
- Collate information on the location of the injured and their condition
- Request the establishment of a Survivor Reception Centre
- Liaise with friends and relatives of casualties and survivors
- Provide conference facilities for briefings or media statements by incident commanders
- May be able to provide a helicopter(s)/drones for the aerial assessment of the scene

4.3 Role of the fire and rescue service at a major incident

The fire and rescue service has a major role in the management of hazards at the scene. As stated previously, they often retain control of the immediate site. The initial responsibilities of the fire and rescue service are given in Box 4.4.

Box 4.4 Fire and rescue service initial responsibilities

- Establishing a Forward Control Point
- Commencing an incident log
- Saving life
- Preventing escalation of the incident
- Extinguishing fires
- Reducing or eliminating hazards
- Extricating trapped casualties
- Clearing routes in and out of the wreckage
- Liaising with other emergency services
- Providing specialist equipment (lighting, lifting, shelters)
- Providing mass decontamination assets under the control of the ambulance service
- Extricating the dead

Fire and rescue service predetermined attendance

The number of fire service vehicles initially dispatched is determined by a risk assessment and is termed the 'predetermined attendance' (PDA).

In any given geographical area, there will be several high-risk areas such as an airport or petrochemical works. These are potential sites for major incidents; with predetermined plans the initial response to a call from such an area is likely be above the standard requirement.

Like other emergency services, the fire and rescue service have several special appliances that are operationally available and that may form part of the PDA to a specific incident.

Duties of the Fire Commander

When a major incident is declared a senior officer is required to take command of the fire and rescue service resources at the scene. The command responsibilities of this officer are shown in Box 4.5.

Box 4.5 Duties of the Fire Commander

- Assume command of all fire and rescue service resources, taking charge of all operations concerned with firefighting, saving life from fire and rescue of trapped persons
- Establish a command post in the control unit near to the Police and Ambulance Control units
- Nominate officers to take charge of various sectors of the incident, and nominate safety officers
- Provide special equipment such as high-volume pumps and rescue equipment
- Where fire is not involved, deploy personnel and equipment in liaison with the Police and Ambulance Commanders, and generally assist the other services
- Provide or obtain specialist assistance where hazardous substances are involved

Two problems may beset the fire and rescue service early in the major incident – access and a continuing supply of water. Access may be difficult if the incident occurs away from a main road (such as on a railway line or in a tunnel). The water carried by a pumping appliance can be rapidly consumed in a severe fire. It is then necessary to take water from hydrants, streams, rivers, ponds and any other sources that are available locally.

Fire and rescue service aid to the health services

The fire and rescue service can assist the medical services at the scene of a major incident as shown in Box 4.6.

Box 4.6 Fire and rescue service aid to the medical services

- Provide a safe area to work by removing fire, chemical, electrical or other hazards and by clearing routes into and out of the immediate scene
- Provide an improved area to work with lighting, shelter and improved access to the trapped patient
- Provide skills and equipment to extricate entrapped casualties
- Provide personnel to lift and carry casualties from the incident to the Casualty Clearing Station
- Provide first aid

4.4 Role of the maritime and coastguard services at a major incident

Maritime and coastguard agencies will have a principal role in coordinating the rescue of casualties from an offshore incident. The initial responsibilities are indicated in Box 4.7.

Box 4.7 Initial responsibilities of the maritime and coastguard agencies

- Coordinating incidents when offshore and in territorial waters
- Plotting the position of the incident
- Broadcasting to alert vessels in the area
- Establishing communication (if possible) with the person in charge to ascertain assistance required and intentions
- Requesting the deployment of air assets immediately to the scene
- Tasking specialists for transport to the vessel/installation (including fire and health services)
- Launching appropriate lifeboat assistance
- Contacting Naval Command for available naval units

4.5 Summary

- The police are usually in control of a major incident
- All emergency services have special responsibilities at a major incident
- All emergency services will assist health services to save lives

CHAPTER 5
Support service organisation and roles

Learning outcomes

After reading this chapter you will be able to:
- List the support services available to assist in a major incident response
- Describe how these agencies can assist the health services at the scene of a major incident

5.1 Introduction

The support services are those agencies that are not part of the health or emergency services that may be requested to provide assistance at the scene of a major incident. They include the following:

- The local civil authority
- Voluntary aid societies
- Voluntary ambulance services (for example, Red Cross, Red Crescent, St John Ambulance Service, St Andrews First Aid)
- The military

5.2 Specific services

Local authority

In the acute phase of a major incident response, a local civil authority can provide assistance to the emergency services and can provide support to the community. In the longer term the local authority will have a primary role in the recovery of the community.

Support to the emergency services

Initially, the response may be to provide machinery and equipment to assist in the rescue operation. Earth-moving equipment may be needed to clear routes, steps may be laid on embankments and additional lighting can be provided. Public transport may be used for casualty evacuation. Shelter may be provided to establish rest centres with provision for food and drinks; those who require temporary accommodation will be housed.

Long-term recovery

Over weeks or months, the local authority will continue to support survivors. Cleansing, environmental health, housing, public works and building departments may all be involved in the restoration of normality for the community.

Major Incident Medical Management and Support: The Practical Approach at the Scene, Fourth Edition.
Edited by Tony Gleeson and Kevin Mackway-Jones.
© 2023 John Wiley & Sons Ltd. Published 2023 by John Wiley & Sons Ltd.

Voluntary aid societies

Voluntary aid societies can provide practical support such as basic life support, humanitarian assistance and victim support. They can also provide support to the emergency responders, for example, hot food/drinks. In the context of a major incident this support for the emergency services and survivors at the scene should not be undervalued.

Voluntary ambulance services

There are voluntary ambulance services in most developed countries. These may be mobilised as part of the health service major incident plan, or by the police following a request from the Ambulance Commander. The aid offered by these services is listed in Box 5.1.

Box 5.1 Aid offered by the voluntary ambulance services

- Staff to resource a first aid post in the Survivor Reception Centre and rest centres
- Transport of patients with minor injuries to definitive care facilities
- Staff for stretcher-bearing duties
- Support to the ambulance service in their 'business as usual' activity

---

In addition, organisations such as the Red Cross, the Red Crescent, St John Ambulance Service, and St Andrew's First Aid can often provide vehicle resources that are able to respond under the direction and direct control of the ambulance service.

Military

Although it requires ministerial approval for deployment, the armed forces are a potential source of additional organised, trained and disciplined personnel. In addition to this simple manpower resource, the armed forces have knowledge, skills and equipment that may be especially useful when the incident is compound (see Chapter 1).

The response by the armed forces may depend upon the geographical location of the incident, the time scale and, most critically, the availability of military personnel and equipment subject to existing operational commitments. With the exception of a few specialist capabilities, the armed forces are generally unable to guarantee a specific response and therefore should not be relied on in civil emergency plans.

Specialist parts of the military can be of specific assistance to the civil community. For example, explosive ordnance disposal (EOD) teams may be required to neutralise any explosive devices or to confirm that devices have been destroyed. Where there is a special risk, such as that posed by a chemical, biological, radiological or nuclear (CBRN) device, the armed forces can provide some expertise in planning and response that would not be available from a civilian source.

5.3 Summary

- Support services are available to complement the regular emergency and health service responses to a major incident

PART III
Preparation

CHAPTER 6
Planning

Learning outcomes

After reading this chapter you will be able to:
- Describe the guidance available for the emergency services and other agencies
- List the specific guidance that exists for the health service
- Describe the structured approach to a response

6.1 Introduction

Although each of the emergency services has different responsibilities and priorities in the event of a major incident, saving life is the primary aim of all agencies. Many other responsibilities are common to all services (Box 6.1). To achieve an efficient response, it is important that multiagency planning, education and exercising have taken place so that each service is aware of the roles and priorities of others. Most international emergency planning guidance explicitly encourages this multiagency approach.

Box 6.1 Combined response objectives

- Save life
- Prevent escalation of the incident
- Relieve suffering
- Protect the environment
- Protect property
- Rapidly restore normality
- Facilitate enquiries

6.2 Guidance

In most countries, major incident guidance is published by the national government. In the UK, for example, guidance is available for England and also for each devolved administration. This guidance may be supplemented by web publications outlining policy and practice, and is often underpinned by statutory responsibilities. More often than not nowadays, major incident response is placed within a framework of business continuity management (BCM). The guidance available allocates responsibility for various necessary functions or services at the scene of the incident to different responding organisations. One such scheme is shown in Table 6.1.

Major Incident Medical Management and Support: The Practical Approach at the Scene, Fourth Edition.
Edited by Tony Gleeson and Kevin Mackway-Jones.
© 2023 John Wiley & Sons Ltd. Published 2023 by John Wiley & Sons Ltd.

Table 6.1 Agency responsibilities

Task	Agency
Care of the uninjured survivor	Police Social services Local authority
Care of the injured survivor	Health service Police Fire service
Dealing with fatalities (identification)	Police
Dealing with fatalities (confirmation)	Health service
Running information centres	Police
Dealing with friends/relatives	Police Social services Local authority Health service
Evacuation and providing temporary shelter	Police Local authority
Social support	Social services Local authority

6.3 General principles

Emergency planning guidance usually requires that an 'all-hazards' approach to planning is adopted by all the services involved. The planning approach must accommodate incidents of major, mass and catastrophic proportion with a variety of causes (Box 6.2). One cannot make assumptions that all major incidents will arise from a traumatic incident with a manageable number of casualties and with no impact on infrastructure. Planning for all potential eventualities must be considered.

Box 6.2 The planning approach

Major	Individual hospitals handle the incident within current and long-established major incident plans. Number of casualties: tens.
Mass	Larger scale incident with possibility of involving the closure or evacuation of a major health facility, or persistent disruption over many days. Collective mutual aid response required from neighbouring hospitals. Number of casualties: hundreds.
Catastrophic	An incident that is of such proportions that it severely disrupts health and social care and other support functions (for example, water, electricity, transport). These are compound incidents. The required response exceeds collective local capacity. Number of casualties: thousands.

Plans must also include arrangements to deal with large numbers of specific injury types, such as major burns, and population groups such as children. In addition, a strategy for protraction (potentially requiring casualty care on scene, extending over many hours or even days) needs to be thought through.

Planning must take place in conjunction with the other agencies involved. A multiagency approach is essential if a cohesive and effective response is to succeed. Both the voluntary sector and (potentially) private sector agencies within the locality need to be fully engaged in the process.

6.4 Incorporating the structured approach into the response

Command and control

Health service command structures and levels need to correlate with those of all the emergency services at the scene of an incident. The standard agreed levels of Strategic (Gold), Tactical (Silver) and Operational (Bronze) are used widely by the health service both at the scene and in hospitals. There is a move away from the Gold, Silver and Bronze nomenclature although you will find them used interchangeably with the newer Strategic, Tactical and Operational terms. It is essential that health service plans incorporate the role and requirements of each level; and detail the command and reporting structures to be followed locally, regionally and nationally.

Safety

Risk assessment and management is encouraged throughout all current guidance and should form the basis for local planning activity. National Risk Registers can be used to identify significant local risks (such as airports, sports stadia, etc.) and these must be assessed and multiagency plans for their management should be developed. Incident-specific plans need to identify clear safety precautions and procedures for staff, together with training requirements.

Communications

Standardised alert messages must be included in all plans and used to avoid any confusion. The plans must clearly identify what these messages are; what response is required when they are received and that staff are aware of them, their meaning and the implications. For example, in stadia there are frequently code words/phrases used and announced over the tannoys to inform staff of the potential for a major incident response. These code phrases are innocuous enough so as not to trigger panic amongst the crowd.

The communications section of plans must also include arrangements for liaison with, and the provision of information to, the Police Casualty Bureau. Media impact should not be underestimated, and media management should be included as a specific subsection of the communications plan.

Assessment

Plans should detail the amount and type of information required by senior officers/staff when scene assessment has been undertaken. Health service commanders should give early warning of any health issues as they arise using the HANE format (see Chapter 14).

Triage

The triage algorithms used in a major incident setting differ from those used in normal health services emergency care. It is essential that plans identify which algorithms are to be used and that, wherever possible, validated and universally accepted systems are used to ensure consistency and accuracy. Staff must be regularly trained in their use to ensure skill retention, although the use of aide memoires for any algorithms not used on standard triage labelling systems should be encouraged.

Treatment

Major incident plans should be based on the premise that the standard of care will mirror the treatment that would be used in normal practice wherever possible. Medical equipment supplied to the scene should match that in regular daily use, although there may also be items specific to mass casualty emergency care. Training for staff should include an awareness of what equipment can be supplied to the scene, how to activate resupply and the scope of the care that should be provided to ensure safe and appropriate initial resuscitation and transfer from the scene.

Transport

Arrangements for the transfer of casualties from the scene to receiving hospitals, and the provision of transport for health staff to the scene, must be clearly stated.

6.5 Recovery

Plans should not only cover the initial response phase of any incident. The recovery phase needs to be considered early during the response, and clear instructions need to be given to ensure that staff can initiate appropriate business continuity arrangements.

The aims are to ensure that normal service provision is resumed as early as is practicable; that staff get the necessary support, rest and recuperation; and that equipment and supplies are replenished promptly. Health service organisations need to consider the impact of the incident on their critical and core services and plan for the medium and long-term staffing, resources and financial needs accordingly.

6.6 Summary

- A multiagency, 'all-hazards' approach to planning for a major incident is essential for a coordinated and effective response
- Plans will only be effective if staff have been appropriately trained and the necessary equipment is provided
- Plans should cover the recovery phase

CHAPTER 7
Personal equipment

Learning outcomes

After reading this chapter you will be able to:
- Describe the minimum safe clothing requirements for pre-hospital health care
- Discuss which additional items of clothing and personal equipment are desirable in order to improve comfort and efficiency

7.1 Minimum clothing

The most important considerations for pre-hospital care clothing are:

- Personal safety
- Function and durability
- Comfort

Personal safety

Personal safety for the rescuers is paramount. Any ambulance or medical personnel attending the scene should be equipped with appropriate personal protective clothing. A doctor in theatre scrubs or a nurse in uniform is a liability both to themselves and to others. Individuals who are inappropriately dressed should be refused entry to the scene. As this may mean turning away potentially useful personnel, compromise may be necessary. If there is a supply of protective clothing carried on the ambulance service equipment vehicle, then appropriate clothing can be issued. Otherwise, these staff may be able to work safely within the confines of the Casualty Clearing Station without the need for full protective equipment.

Key point

Individuals who are inappropriately dressed should be denied access to the site.

The responsibility for the safety of all health service personnel at the scene is delegated to the Ambulance Safety Officer. Medical teams will usually arrive at the Ambulance Parking Point, which is an appropriate place to check personal protective equipment.

Personal safety implies protection against predictable hazards. The hazards and their solutions are listed in Table 7.1.

Major Incident Medical Management and Support: The Practical Approach at the Scene, Fourth Edition.
Edited by Tony Gleeson and Kevin Mackway-Jones.
© 2023 John Wiley & Sons Ltd. Published 2023 by John Wiley & Sons Ltd.

Table 7.1 Protective clothing solutions for predictable hazards

Hazard	Protective clothing solution
Emergency vehicles	High visibility jacket or tabard
Elements (rain, wind, snow)	Waterproof and insulated full body protection
Injury to head	Hard hat with three-point chinstrap
Injury to eyes	Safety glasses or goggles, or visor
Injury to face	Visor
Noise	Ear defenders
Injury to hands	Heavy duty gloves (debris gloves)
Blood and body fluid exposure	Standard clinical precaution and equipment
Injury to feet	Heavy duty oil- and acid-resistant boots with protective toecaps

Function and durability

Visibility

A high-visibility reflective jacket or tabard should be worn. For the ambulance service these will normally be green and yellow as recommended in the international identifications policy.

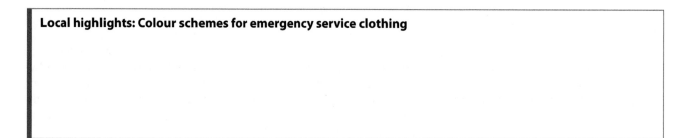

Local highlights: Colour schemes for emergency service clothing

Identification

The jacket or tabard should be clearly labelled on the front and back and read 'Doctor' or 'Nurse' for medical staff. Ambulance staff may use 'Ambulance' or 'Paramedic'.

Health service commanders should be separately identified. The Senior Ambulance Officer on scene wears a green and white chequered tabard labelled 'Ambulance Commander' (or local term). The Senior Clinician on scene wears a conventional tabard labelled 'Doctor' (or local term). The colour of lettering for all health service name banners is green on white.

It may also be useful for staff in other key appointments to be clearly labelled with tabards to enable identification from a distance.

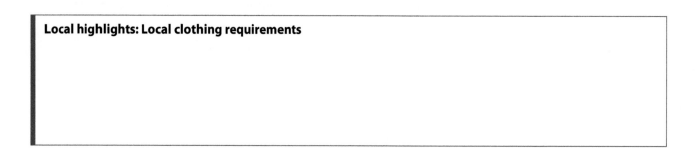

Local highlights: Local clothing requirements

> **Key point**
>
> Standardisation of clothing is important to prevent confusion between emergency service personnel, and to aid identification from a distance.

Warmth and waterproofing

In cold weather warm underclothing is important. This is particularly an issue for staff deployed from hospital who may wear a jacket and over-trousers on top of their everyday working clothes. In hot weather a balance of visibility and protection against potential heat stress is necessary and flexibility is required and layers of protective clothing should be available.

> **Key point**
>
> In hot climates a degree of protection may have to be sacrificed for comfort.

Protection against injury

A hard hat is mandatory. Hats have the tendency to fall off and a helmet that has a secure chin strap (three-point strap) is recommended. The helmet should be of high specification (for example, Kevlar® composite). A torch can be mounted on the helmet, which will allow both hands to remain free. The colour of both the helmet and any lettering may be specified.

> **Local highlights: Helmet markings and colours**

A visor is required to protect the face and, unless it is close fitting, separate goggles or safety glasses must protect the eyes independently. Ear defenders are required to protect the ears from the background noise. These can be fitted to the helmet or carried separately. Both a heavy-duty pair of gloves (to protect against glass and sharp metal) and patient treatment gloves (to protect against blood) are needed. Strong, correctly fitting footwear with metal toecaps are needed. Boots should also be oil and acid resistant. Wellington boots are commonly stocked by hospitals for pre-hospital use but must be of high specification if they are to fulfil the requirements of a major incident scene and may be inappropriate for walking on uneven ground.

Chemical resistance

It must be possible to protect health service personnel in a chemical environment. This requires additional training to use the necessary personal protective equipment, which will invariably include a respirator with a chemical filter. Special incidents are discussed in more detail in Part VI.

Equipment storage

Clothing should have enough pockets to store essential personal items.

Durability

Some protective clothing is reinforced at the knee and elbow. This is useful when working on the floor. The fabric must be durable against rip hazards at the scene. Again, there may need to be a compromise in hot climates between durability and comfort.

Fire-retardant properties

Basic standards of fire retardancy should be specified in all protective clothing for the health services.

Comfort

If clothing is not issued on a personal basis, then a range of sizes of personal protective equipment must be available. Potential responders should make sure they have tried on the clothing in training prior to mobilisation so they can quickly find the size that fits them.

7.2 Additional items

Additional items of personal equipment that may be carried are detailed in this section.

Personal identification

This is essential for any staff who travel independently to the scene since access may be denied if they are unable to prove their identity. It is less critical for staff arriving in marked emergency vehicles, though still desirable.

Mobile phone

The use of mobile phones at the scene of a major incident will be unavoidable and, in some circumstances, may be more important for commanders than a radio (see Chapter 13). A spare battery is useful.

Notebook

A log of actions and events is essential. Not only will it aid confirmation that requests for assistance have been actioned, but it is increasingly necessary to justify decisions in the setting of the inevitable public inquiry. Any notes made must be kept.

Recording devices

Some individuals prefer a dictaphone to a notebook. While this may be faster to record, it is more difficult to review the entries and background noise may mask the dictation. They can however be very helpful when reviewing decisions post the event and when writing your incident logbook. Rather than clicking on and off, some individuals just start it and leave it recording during the incident, changing tapes as required. This will capture interactions with other services and the shared decision making between services which may be critical in the post incident review.

Aide-memoires and action cards

All personnel in key health service appointments should be provided with action cards listing their responsibilities. Commercially designed, waterproof, major incident aide-memoires are available.

Camera

It is not a legal requirement to obtain consent before photography for evidence or communication purposes and any photograph taken should be available for investigation and legal proceedings. A photograph can accompany a patient to hospital if this will help in their further management (it may assist the hospital staff appreciate the mechanism and severity of an injury).

Torch

A helmet torch is recommended.

Whistle

A whistle is commonly employed by the fire service to indicate an escalating threat requiring immediate evacuation. This generally precludes its use by other personnel.

Money and credit or debit cards

It is unlikely that there will be any charge for refreshments at the scene for working staff, but doctors and nurses can find themselves stranded in a distant hospital if they have acted as an escort for an individual patient. Even in a major incident, they may need to cover their own expenses.

Incident management system

Commercially available incident management systems have been used by civilian and military personnel. They are often contained in a specially designed rucksack and may include:

- Packs of triage labels, with an algorithm for the triage sieve (see Chapter 15) and a tally card of patients triaged
- Incident sketch board and casualty state board
- Major incident aide-memoire
- Camera
- Recording devices
- Torch and chemi-luminescent light sticks
- Tabards for key appointments (Senior Ambulance Officer on scene, Triage)
- Field rations for one and water bottle
- Local maps

Computer

Computer-based management support systems with the potential for online remote advice have been developed, and this level of technology is currently being used.

7.3 Summary

- All health service staff must adhere to minimum clothing requirements
- The health service senior officers (or delegated representative) should refuse entry to the scene of any personnel who are incorrectly dressed
- Clothing colours should conform to national standards and conventions in order to aid recognition and prevent confusion
- Clothing should be functional, durable and comfortable, but above all should provide protection against the predictable hazards
- The basic requirements may be enhanced by a number of additional items of personal equipment

CHAPTER 8
Medical equipment

Learning outcomes

After reading this chapter you will be able to:
- Describe why extra medical equipment is necessary
- List the equipment required for triage, first aid or advanced life support
- List the equipment required for specialist medical skills by medical teams
- List the equipment required when packaging for transport
- Discuss the best way to store equipment
- Define how medical equipment is resupplied to the scene
- Discuss the role of the Ambulance Equipment Officer

8.1 Introduction

Like all aspects of major incident care, the provision of medical equipment requires forward planning. Equipment requirements are different from normal pre-hospital care for two main reasons. First, the number of casualties will be much larger than under normal circumstances. Second, the time elapsed before casualties arrive at hospital (and therefore the time spent on scene providing treatment) may be greatly increased. This is not only due to entrapment, but also because casualty numbers can exceed the transport capacity for evacuation. Emergency ambulances deployed to a major incident will have insufficient equipment to treat all the casualties and therefore extra provision must be made by the ambulance service and any attending medical teams. Ambulance services may consider a predetermined attendance (PDA) which will ensure a certain amount of vehicles, officers and equipment will be sent as standard to the scene on the declaration of a major incident.

Key point

Extra equipment must be provided by both the ambulance service and individual medical teams.

8.2 Levels of medical intervention

The equipment provided to support a major incident should reflect the levels of intervention that are available. There are five levels of medical intervention at the scene:

1. Triage.
2. Life-saving first aid.
3. Advanced life support.
4. Specialist medical support.
5. Packaging for transport.

Major Incident Medical Management and Support: The Practical Approach at the Scene, Fourth Edition.
Edited by Tony Gleeson and Kevin Mackway-Jones.
© 2023 John Wiley & Sons Ltd. Published 2023 by John Wiley & Sons Ltd.

Triage

Proper performance of triage requires both a triage system to be in place and a labelling system to indicate that triage has been performed. Triage labels should be easily and securely attached to the patient, must be marked and colour coded for priority, must be durable and weather resistant but still be able to be written on and must facilitate rapid and clear re-categorisation. Folding triage labels best fit this specification. Triage labels should be carried on all emergency ambulances so that there is no delay in initiating this process. Triage is discussed in detail in Chapter 15.

Key point

Triage labels are required on each emergency ambulance.

Special equipment may be necessary to encourage appropriate triage of children.

Life-saving first aid

The type of equipment used for first aid is similar to that used by the ambulance service on a day-to-day basis. The principal difference in a major incident is the quantity that will be required. Equipment should allow immediate intervention in life-threatening conditions affecting the airway, breathing or circulation (ABC). The equipment requirements for life-saving first aid are listed in Table 8.1.

Table 8.1 Equipment to support life-saving first aid

Intervention	Equipment
Control of catastrophic haemorrhage	Dressings Tourniquet
Clear the airway	Manual suction apparatus
Maintain the airway	Oropharyngeal airway Nasopharyngeal airway
Support ventilation	Face shield Pocket mask Bag and mask
Seal open pneumothorax	Chest seal
Arrest compressible haemorrhage	Absorbent pressure dressings

It is debatable whether equipment should be provided to support ventilation in the first aid phase. If a major incident casualty fails to breathe after the airway has been opened, the triage sieve will categorise the patient as 'dead'. However, particular circumstances may arise where a more active approach is appropriate. Considerations include the type of injury, the number of casualties, number of responders, access to hospital and age of the patient. Judgement will be required. In general however, in large incidents, deviation from the triage sieve categorisation will have a detrimental effect on overall patient outcomes and will prevent doing the 'most for the most'.

Local highlights: Life-saving first aid

> **Key point**
>
> First aid requires simple equipment to support life-threatening conditions affecting the airway, breathing or circulation.

Advanced life support

Advanced life support will predominantly be provided at the Casualty Clearing Station (CCS), although some interventions will be required on site for trapped patients. The equipment needs of the CCS are familiar to those who work in emergency medicine, since the main requirement is for resources to stabilise the ABCs. There are a number of ways of arranging the supply and resupply of this area.

One way is to arrange items in patient sets with one complete set of equipment for the control of ABC per patient. In this scheme a primary treatment box or rucksack stays by each patient and equipment is consequently close at hand if required urgently. Although this system will result in a degree of overprovision, it avoids the confusion that can arise when searching for equipment from a central storage area. Resupply is simple because the set of equipment can be returned to the equipment vehicle for replenishment once the casualty leaves the scene.

An alternative scheme is to keep non-disposable items (such as self-inflating bags and laryngoscopes) in a central area, and issue boxes or rucksacks of disposable items (such as dressings, airways, intravenous cannulas and fluids) either in single or multi-patient packs. This avoids the problem of supplying expensive items to each individual casualty area. Resupply of the disposable item sets is from a central store.

The additional equipment requirements for advanced life support are listed in Table 8.2. All the capabilities listed in first aid can also be delivered at the advanced life support level.

As previously discussed, equipment to support breathing may not be needed but is usually carried. The underlying dilemma is that the use of limited resources to support a continuing need for ventilation in an individual may not be in the best interest of the majority.

It is unlikely that there will be sufficient resources to treat cardiac arrest at the site. Where cardiac arrest occurs in the CCS it is appropriate to follow treatment algorithms, including defibrillation where resources allow, but the patient load may dictate the final extent of the resuscitation attempt.

Table 8.2 Additional equipment to support advanced life support

Intervention	Equipment
Secure the airway	Supraglottic airway device (LMA or iGel) Endotracheal tube
Deliver oxygen	Portable oxygen source and mask with reservoir delivery system for spontaneously breathing patients
Support ventilation	Bag–valve–mask set
Decompress tension pneumothorax	Needle for thoracocentesis
Splintage for haemorrhage control	Traction splint
Spinal immobilisation	Semi-rigid cervical collar Long spinal board
Replace fluid volume	Intravenous cannula and fluid Intraosseous needle
Relief of pain	Simple splint Entonox Analgesics Burns dressings, for example, cling film

Spinal immobilisation should be reserved for high-risk patients. Precautionary immobilisation for mechanism alone will be inappropriate where several hundred patients may have been exposed to the same mechanism (for example, a high-energy train crash). Equipment for spinal immobilisation will normally be carried by the individual ambulance or helicopter transporting the patient to hospital.

Equipment must also be supplied to treat any children involved in a major incident. The paediatric triage tape along with colour-coded packs of equipment according to weight may enable rapid selection of the appropriate size of equipment for the child.

Where any sharps are to be used for clinical care, facilities for safe disposal must be available.

Local highlights: Equipment needed for extended paramedic skills

---

Specialist medical support

Any medical team must supply the equipment necessary for advanced procedures not normally performed by paramedics. Their equipment must supplement that carried by the ambulance service rather than duplicate it. It is also important that any medical team equipment is compatible with that supplied by the ambulance service.

Key point

Medical team equipment should be compatible with ambulance service equipment. It should supplement rather than duplicate, and must reflect the extended skills of the team.

Medical teams will usually carry their own equipment to the scene, but may make arrangements for it to be stored by the ambulance service in equipment vehicles. Any medical team should be prepared to undertake the procedures that are likely to be required in the first hour of on-site care. Of particular importance is the need to carry sufficient analgesia for parenteral administration, appropriate drugs for sedation for procedures on, or extrication of, trapped patients and local anaesthetic agents for use in regional blocks. It is important that the contents of the equipment containers for the major incident medical teams are clearly distinguishable from those used for day-to-day pre-hospital work. This can be achieved either by appropriate written marking or by using a different colour of container. Overall, it is probably better to have a single system for use in both circumstances since the response is more likely to be effective in a crisis when individuals are familiar with the organisation and content of equipment.

The *additional* equipment requirements for specialist medical support are listed in Table 8.3. All the capabilities listed in 'first aid' and 'advanced aid' can also be delivered at the specialist medical level.

Table 8.3 Additional equipment to support the medical team

Intervention	Equipment
Secure the airway	Surgical cricothyroidotomy
Support ventilation	Automatic ventilator Chest drain set with drainage bag
Treat cardiac disease	12 lead electrocardiograms External pacing
Replace fluid volume	Rapid infusion device/pressure infuser Adult/paediatric intraosseous device
Amputate/disarticulate limb	Amputation set
Advanced drugs	Drug-assisted intubation and maintenance of anaesthesia Anaesthesia, local Analgesia, intravenous Sedation, intravenous or intramuscular Medical emergencies Cardiac arrest

In some areas the responsibility for medical care at major incidents may rest with voluntary immediate-care doctors. They usually only carry equipment for the treatment of a relatively small number of casualties. In such circumstances, arrangements may need to be made with local hospitals or with the ambulance service to supply equipment that would otherwise be brought by the hospital-based medical teams.

Packaging for transport

Patients must be packaged for transport prior to leaving the scene for hospital and additional equipment may be required for this. Examples are listed in Table 8.4.

Table 8.4 Additional equipment to support packaging for transport

Intervention	Equipment
Secure intravenous cannulas	Splints
Immobilise fractured femur	Traction splint
Spinal immobilisation	Vacuum mattress

Where rigid spinal immobilisation is required, and particularly where there is a delay in transfer to hospital for clinical spinal injury, it may be preferable to immobilise the patient within a vacuum mattress rather than on a long spinal board. This may reduce the likelihood of developing pressure sores.

8.3 Equipment containers

Various types of container can be considered to carry medical equipment. Key factors in choosing the design are:

- Ease with which they can be carried over uneven terrain and over long distances (rucksacks are suited to this and leave both hands free to assist in movement)
- Ease with which contents can be accessed (top loading where access to equipment at the bottom requires all other equipment to be removed first is not a good solution, while rucksacks that have multiple pockets/pouches with clear fronts are popular)
- Security of the contents (if you drop the container, it does not spill its contents)
- Visibility (if you put it down, you can find it again)

> **Key point**
>
> Containers should be easy to carry and keep equipment visible, accessible and secure.

All potential users have a responsibility to be familiar with the equipment and the way it is stored. Regular checking of the equipment by the staff that will use it or regular use in training improves familiarity.

Standardisation of equipment sets is desirable as a number of different organisations will often share equipment in a major incident.

> **Key point**
>
> Standardisation of equipment allows interoperability between rescuers and easy resupply.

The best arrangement is to have a universally agreed type of equipment bag organised in a standard manner. All personnel can use this, and should supplies run short, a full bag can be delivered. Ideally, major incident equipment sets should be standardised nationally.

The actual equipment provided for a major incident needs to be agreed on at regional level as it will depend on:

- The predefined capabilities of the attending clinicians in terms of clinical skills provided
- The anticipated clinical capacity of the health services on the scene

8.4 Equipment resupply

Resupply by the ambulance service

Each ambulance service must plan to rapidly deploy additional equipment to the scene of a major incident; most have one or more equipment vehicles ('emergency/incident support units') for this purpose. The exact number and distribution of these varies but in the UK many services would aim to have the equipment vehicle to the scene within 20 minutes.

Some services use trailer units, whilst others use specifically designed vehicles. Local conditions will determine which is most appropriate. Whatever the design, it is important that the vehicle is clearly marked as the central equipment supply.

Equipment carried on these units will resupply triage, first aid and advanced life support capabilities. The exact amount of equipment that should be made available depends on both the incidents that might occur and the number of vehicles deployed. In the case of prolonged incidents, arrangements must be made for additional supplies to be brought to the scene either by replenishing the equipment vehicle or by replacing them.

In addition to resupply of disposable medical supplies the equipment vehicle is likely to carry:

- Portable shelter, with a heating system in appropriate climates
- Portable lighting with generator
- Signs ('Casualty Clearing Station', 'Parking Point', 'Loading Point', etc.)
- Folding stretchers
- Blankets
- Oxygen resupply with multiple valve outlets

Occasionally, an unexpected clinical procedure may be necessary. In this circumstance, the Senior Clinician on scene will need to make contact with a local hospital to arrange the supply of the equipment or drug. Ideally, prearranged procedures should be in place to guarantee the timely delivery of the correct item to the correct person.

As medical teams are rotated, further specialist medical equipment will be brought to the scene. Rucksacks can be very similar and should be clearly identified by the name of the hospital or organisation. This will ensure the return of all equipment sets to the right unit following the incident.

Blood

Blood will only be required at scene in exceptional circumstances. The Senior Clinician on scene should liaise with the local blood transfusion services. If a facility for donation is required this would normally be established at regular donor centres.

Supply from national stocks

In many countries strategically located stocks of equipment are maintained for use in the event of a major incident or mass casualty situation. Plans should include the ability to rapidly deploy this equipment to the site following a request to the Ambulance Control Centre.

This equipment may include:

- ABC equipment for resuscitation, plus mass wound and burns dressings
- Modesty equipment for patients post chemical decontamination, for example, paper suits and space blankets
- Antidotes, treatments and vaccine for specific chemical, biological, nerve and poisoning agents

Resources may also be supplemented by mutual aid from other regions and organisations.

8.5 Equipment Officer

If there is more than one equipment vehicle at the scene, it is important that an ambulance officer is designated as the Ambulance Equipment Officer. Medical teams may leave their resupply and surplus specialist equipment with this officer.

> **Key point**
>
> An Ambulance Equipment Officer should be nominated to ensure the appropriate use of stores.

The Ambulance Equipment Officer must ensure that stores are issued appropriately and in a controlled fashion. Certain items (such as the Senior Ambulance Officer's on-scene tabard) must be strictly controlled if a scene is to be effectively managed. Other items (such as drugs) should only be issued to appropriately qualified and trained staff. If more than one equipment vehicle is present, then only one vehicle should be used at a time; this facilitates resupply as the other vehicle can then be sent for restocking once empty.

The Ambulance Equipment Officer's most difficult task is ensuring that equipment supply is coordinated. Several requests may arrive from varying sources for the same equipment for one patient, leading to waste. On other occasions equipment can get diverted en route.

8.6 Summary

- Extra equipment will be necessary to deal with major incidents
- This equipment is required for triage, first aid, advanced life support and packaging for transport
- The ambulance service will usually provide equipment vehicles at the scene and should also nominate an Ambulance Equipment Officer to coordinate distribution and resupply
- Medical teams should bring their own specialist equipment to the scene for advanced procedures
- Any equipment stored for use in the event of a major incident should be regularly checked, serviced and used in practice scenarios by the potential users
- Equipment resupply may occur from the ambulance service, from hospitals or from predetermined national stocks

CHAPTER 9
Training

Learning outcomes

After reading this chapter you will be able to:
- Describe the place of MIMMS education in health emergency planning
- List the range of exercises used to support major incident education

9.1 Introduction

Working in a pre-hospital environment requires specialist knowledge and skills. Coupled with this, the stress associated with responding to a major incident can be challenging for individuals. However, major incidents are (fortunately) infrequent occurrences. Very few health service personnel will be involved in such an event more than once or twice during their career. In such circumstances, training becomes very important. As in all areas, good performance must be built on sound foundations. The *Major Incident Medical Management and Support* (MIMMS) approach provides this.

9.2 Education

The MIMMS principles are the fundamental building blocks for major incident education (Figure 9.1). They can be enhanced by practical skills training, table-top exercises and practical exercises without casualties (PEWCs), progressing to single service exercises and ultimately multiagency exercises with casualties.

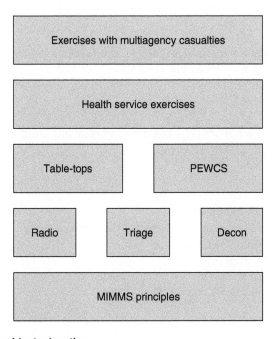

Figure 9.1 Building blocks of major incident education

Major Incident Medical Management and Support: The Practical Approach at the Scene, Fourth Edition.
Edited by Tony Gleeson and Kevin Mackway-Jones.
© 2023 John Wiley & Sons Ltd. Published 2023 by John Wiley & Sons Ltd.

MIMMS provides a structured educational approach for Senior Ambulance Officers and Senior Clinicians on scene. It can also provide valuable education about the pre-hospital environment at a major incident scene for hospital staff likely to be deployed to an incident. The 3-day and 2-day advanced MIMMS course delivers specific education and assessment at both Operational and Tactical Commander level. Education for wider roles and processes in major incident planning and delivery should also be to accredited standards and integrated into an educational emergency planning governance programme for health organisations.

Completion of a MIMMS course alone does not fulfil all requirements for health service major incident training. Each health organisation will have a complete programme of continuing professional development (CPD) and every opportunity must be taken to participate in exercises to practically apply and develop those skills.

Exercises

Organisations should consider two broad types of training:

- Emergency preparedness – training key staff to carry out risk assessment, business continuity management (BCM) and emergency planning
- Emergency response – training staff to carry out response functions when an emergency occurs

In most domains, emergency services have a statutory obligation to test and validate emergency plans and procedures. This can be done by exercising.

Three distinct types of exercises have been identified and are as follows:

- A *discussion-based* exercise – they can be used at the policy formulation stage as a 'talk-through' of how to finalise the plan
- A *table-top* multiagency exercise – this type of exercise is particularly useful for validation purposes, particularly for exploring weaknesses in procedures. Table-top exercises are relatively cheap to run, except in the use of staff time
- A major *live* multiagency exercise – requiring a relatively large degree of commitment and possibly funding from a number of organisations

Exercises may be designed to address the needs of a single agency but may require limited input from another agency or agencies.

It is important that all exercise participants undertake an internal organisational debrief, identifying and recording all areas of good practice and those areas that require improvement. In addition, leads from each participating agency need to undertake a multiagency debrief and follow the same process. All lessons learned from these exercises should be fed back into plans and procedures and retested in future exercises.

It is recommended that healthcare organisations carry out a communications exercise at least every 6 months, a table-top exercise at least every year and a live exercise every 3 years.

9.3 Summary

- MIMMS principles underpin major incident education
- MIMMS courses are available and are appropriate for staff in the health services
- Continuing education beyond MIMMS is essential
- Various levels of major incident exercise exist
- Different types of exercise are appropriate for different educational needs
- Lessons learnt from exercises should be incorporated into plans

PART IV
Management

CHAPTER 10
Command and control

Learning outcomes

After reading this chapter you will be able to:
- Define command and control
- Discuss who has overall control at the incident
- Describe the purpose of the cordons at the incident
- List the tiers of command at the incident
- Appreciate the importance of a chain of command with each service

10.1 Introduction

When faced with the chaotic scene of a major incident it is important that order is brought about rapidly. Order requires effective command and control.

Command

Command is the vertical line of authority within each emergency and support service. *Each service has one individual who is in command.* At the scene of the incident, commanders for each of the services are in command of their service.

Control

Control is a horizontal line of authority to direct resources/tasks that may not necessarily be under your command, for example the ambulance service directing fire personnel regarding priority for extrication of casualties. The incident generally has one individual who is in overall control at the scene. This is usually the Police Incident Commander but this will depend on jurisdiction.

By working together to understand the risks associated with the response and having a shared situational awareness of these risks, the commanders can identify the priorities in the response, what options they have in providing the response and how the response is going to be coordinated.

> **Key point**
>
> Command and control are the cornerstones of effective major incident management.

10.2 Incident command

Each service at the scene will have a commander and they will be identified by a distinctive major incident tabard.

The officer in charge of each emergency service on site is referred to as the 'Commander'. Each should wear a distinctive chequered tabard inscribed front and back with their appointment, for example 'Police Incident Commander' (Table 10.1).

Major Incident Medical Management and Support: The Practical Approach at the Scene, Fourth Edition.
Edited by Tony Gleeson and Kevin Mackway-Jones.
© 2023 John Wiley & Sons Ltd. Published 2023 by John Wiley & Sons Ltd.

Table 10.1 Incident commander identifications	
Appointment	**Identifying tabard**
Police Commander	Blue and white chequered
Fire Commander	Red and white chequered
Ambulance Incident Commander	Green and white chequered
Medical Advisor	Green and white chequered

The health service response is led by a single individual who is usually the Ambulance Incident Commander and is supported in the role by the Medical Advisor, usually a doctor with pre-hospital experience and knowledge. The Medical Advisor role is to determine clinical priorities and the appropriate distribution of casualties to places of definitive care. In certain jurisdictions the doctor may be the overall health incident commander and would be called the Medical *Incident* Commander in this case. The actions undertaken by the Medical Advisor are the same as those of the Medical Incident Commander, but the overall legal responsibility for the incident lies with the Ambulance Commander.

Irrespective of whether the ambulance lead or the medical lead takes the overall responsibility for the health response at the scene, it is important that one individual is identified to take the lead on the overall health response at the scene, with the other providing support and advice. Both roles complement each other and, irrespective of who takes overall lead, are essential.

These two officers liaise closely with each other and with the commanders from the fire and police services. The particular title of these commanders will vary from country to country.

The Ambulance Incident Commander and Medical Advisor have distinct roles but must work as a command team. If they work together, efforts will not be duplicated, orders will not be contradictory, troublesome communications will be kept to a minimum and difficult decisions will be shared. If conflict arises, this will be to the detriment of the casualties and potential safety compromises for health service responders.

In the UK there has historically been a reluctance to state the relative positions of the Ambulance and Medical Advisors. However, as the ambulance service has statutory responsibility, the Ambulance Incident Commander can be said to be *in control* of the health services response.

Local highlights: Incident Commander name and identification

Forward Incident Operational (Bronze) Commanders are responsible to the Tactical Incident (Silver) Commander for the management of resources at a specific sector/operational area. The Forward Incident Commander works in a forward operational area/sector and is the 'eyes and ears' of the Tactical Incident Commander. There is a Forward Incident Commander for each designated sector/operational area.

Commanders will focus on a number of function areas in order to meet the organisational responsibilities, these may include:

- Communications
- Fuel resupply
- Mortuary affairs
- Public messaging
- Search and rescue
- Decontamination
- Law enforcement

- Planning support
- Public safety and health
- Emergency medical services
- Mass care

The first vehicle for each service at the scene will initially act as its Incident Control Point. This vehicle should leave its blue lights flashing to identify its role. All other vehicles should extinguish their blue lights. Experience has shown that where this does not happen there can be confusion about where staff report to on arrival.

Each service will have provision for a dedicated incident command vehicle that will carry additional communications equipment and may have briefing facilities. This will take over from the first vehicle on the scene once it arrives.

10.3 Incident control

One service at the scene will have overall responsibility for the effective coordination of the incident. This service should view itself as a facilitator of the other emergency services and ensure close communication and cooperation between them.

In the UK, the police have this responsibility except where an incident occurs 'offshore', where the responsibility rests with the maritime and coastguard agency. In some European countries, for example Sweden, the fire service has overall control. In most countries, in the presence of fire, chemicals or other hazards, the fire service will assume control of the immediate area around the incident (the operational zone within the inner cordon), but the police will still have overall control. Experience in Australia has led to the concept of overall authority resting with the most appropriate agency for the specific type of incident. The so-called 'combat agency' for a conventional man-made major incident would be the police. In the case of a flood the state emergency service would assume control, whilst for an extensive bush fire the fire service would take the role.

It is essential that commanders co-locate and meet regularly where possible to ensure there is a joint strategy in dealing with any incident. This has been proven to mitigate many lessons identified in previous incidents resulting in poor coordination, poor communication, duplication of effort, agencies working in silos and, more importantly, impact on casualty care.

In the UK, through a joint initiative called the Joint Emergency Service Interoperability Principles (JESIP), the emergency services share multiagency command training and organisational major incident terminology (for example, METHANE) eventually publishing them as principles through a joint doctrine. In addition, they adopt a shared decision-making tool (Joint Decision Model or JDM) to support their joint strategy with the aims of saving lives and reducing harm (Figure 10.1).

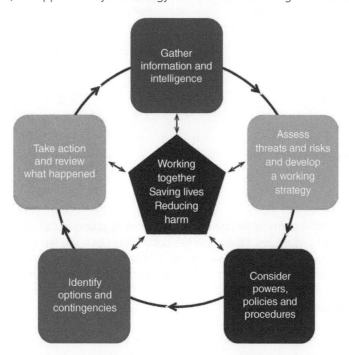

Figure 10.1 Joint Emergency Service Interoperability Principles (JESIP) Joint Decision Model
Reproduced with permission of JESIP

10.4 Cordons

The command and control of any major incident relies on a coordinated, integrated multiagency approach. The police will normally provide coordination of this combined response. A key part of this coordination function is the support of the movement of emergency services to and from the incident. To facilitate this, cordons are put in place. Cordons also prevent anyone without an active role in the incident from gaining access to potentially hazardous areas.

Inner cordon

The *inner cordon* is not always clearly marked unless there is a specific hazard or a scene of crime when it may be denoted by tape. Where a hazard does exist, there may be strict access control across the cordon. In order to ensure complete evacuation if the hazard escalates, individuals must be recorded as going in and going out. Control of movement through the inner cordon may rest with the fire or police service depending on the nature of the hazard.

Outer cordon

The police will determine the extent and location of the outer cordon with the aim of preventing unauthorised access to those areas being used by all services/agencies in relation to the incident.

The police are also responsible for physically establishing the cordon using barrier tape, signs and roadblocks as necessary. Once it is established, only authorised personnel should be allowed through. All vehicles that cross the outer cordon should be clearly marked and all staff should carry personal identification. Medical personnel may attend in unmarked vehicles and may not be able to access the site without personal identification. The cordons are illustrated in Figure 10.2.

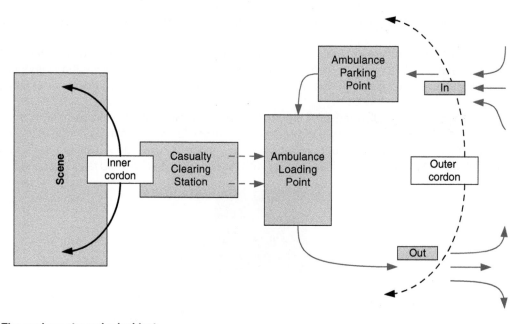

Figure 10.2 The cordons at a major incident

Incident zones

In some major incidents (for example, chemical release or acts of terrorism) access to casualties will be limited to those with specialist training, equipment and procedures. Whilst this has commonly been the fire service, some ambulance services have developed a response capability for hazardous area access (Hazardous Area Response Teams, sometimes called HART teams). These capabilities have been proven to save many lives as the care of casualties starts at the point of patient access.

Some examples of these capabilities are:

- Safe working at height
- Swift water rescue
- Casualty decontamination

- Working in confined spaces
- Tactical medicine (firearms related incidents)
- Self-contained breathing apparatus

Due to the severity of risk in many of these scenarios, the areas (Figure 10.3) defined for a controlled access would be named:

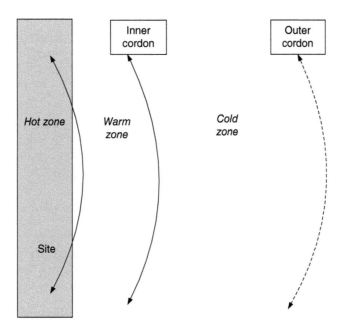

Figure 10.3 Incident zones

Hot zone: The point of immediate danger such as the chemical spillage or currently active discharge of firearms. Only responders with a requirement to deal with the immediate risk/threat should be granted access. This could be fire service controlling a chemical leak or police, or other agency, dealing with a perpetrator.

Warm zone: An area still of significant hazard but out of the way of immediate danger, for example downwind of the chemical plume or no visual sign of active shooter. Access to this area can be granted to specialist ambulance resources.

Both the above can be defined as being within the inner cordon.

Cold zone: An area where the hazard has been sufficiently removed to allow all health service responders (with appropriate levels of personal protective equipment) to access. This is the same as the area within the outer cordon.

Fast moving incidents

The recent experience of incidents involving terrorist activity, for example firearms, knife attacks, using vehicles as a weapon, etc., has generated the need to rethink effective scene management. The generation of multiple scenes and potential terrorist activity remaining in the locale requires a whole new approach to casualty triage, extrication and response.

In such scenarios, only responders who are appropriately trained and protected may enter the hostile areas. Seriously injured casualties are treated with the minimum life-saving techniques, such as control of catastrophic haemorrhage, and then removed to a Casualty Collection Point (CCP) where they will be re-triaged and moved to the Casualty Clearing Station under normal major incident protocols.

10.5 Tiers of command

Various levels of command/management will need to be established to ensure effective control by each emergency service/agency. These levels are nationally agreed and are as follows.

Strategic command

For a 'routine' major incident, there is only one Strategic level of command. In practice it is likely that a Strategic Commander from each agency will coordinate via a Strategic Coordination Group. However, in incidents that cross police force or county boundaries there is a probability that there will be a multiagency Strategic Coordination Group established in each domain. On these occasions it may be decided to establish regional or national coordination.

The Strategic level of command is sometimes referred to as 'Gold' or 'Gold Command(er)'.

A Strategic Commander's purpose is to establish a strategic framework of policy within which a Tactical command can work, thus providing support to the Tactical command and determining plans for the return to a state of normality once the incident is brought under control. The Strategic area is a theoretical boundary beyond the scene, representing a level of senior command that will decide on the resources (physical, human, financial) to assist the scene and business continuity.

Tactical command

The outer cordon encloses the area of responsibility of the incident commanders. This is the Tactical area. The commanders at an incident are in overall command of the scene, allocating resources to the Operational Commanders, planning and coordinating the overall response and obtaining additional resources as necessary.

The Tactical level of command is sometimes referred to as 'Silver' or 'Silver Command(er)'.

The command vehicle for each emergency service may co-locate to form the Joint Emergency Services Control Centre (JESCC), or the Tactical Coordination Centre. For a conventional man-made incident (for example, train crash or terrorist bomb) there is only one Tactical area. For widespread public disorder or a natural occurrence (for example, an earthquake with major structural collapse) there may be two or more discreet major incidents, each regarded as a Tactical area.

It is the responsibility of Tactical Commanders to create a working strategy and a tactical plan and work within the strategy for the incident set by the Strategic Commander.

In conjunction with CSCATTT the following activities are used to develop the tactical plan and incident objectives:

- Determine what has to be done to implement a strategy and what method(s) are likely to achieve success
- Develop a list of resources (personnel, teams, equipment, supplies, facilities) that are required
- Provide a list of resources available
- Compare the resources required with resources available and discuss the findings with the Operational Commanders prior to the operations/tactics meeting
- Draft the tactical plan based on this analysis

Operational command

Operational areas are usually at the site of the incident. Within a Tactical area, there can be any number of Operational areas or *sectors*. Each sector will represent a focus of activity and may require its own Operational Commander. The tiers of command are illustrated in Figure 10.4.

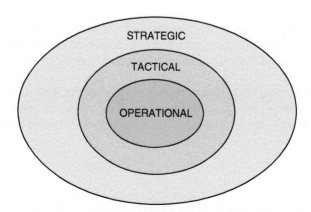

Figure 10.4 The tiers of command

The Operational level of command is sometimes referred to as 'Bronze' or 'Bronze Command(er)'.

Once the tactical plan has been developed and the requisite resources identified, Operational Commanders select specific resources to perform specific work assignments. They should record work assignments/actions in order to report back on delivery and gaps in the tactical plan. Ambulance services will have a number of functional roles at the Operational level of command including parking, primary triage coordination, loading of patients, safety, equipment, etc. This structure can be 'flexed' as needed for the incident requirements.

10.6 The chain of command

Each service has a vertical chain of command at the scene. It is not desirable for command to repeatedly change hands as more senior officers assist as this will interrupt the continuity of management. Ideally, command should change hands once only from the acting commander (in the case of the ambulance service, this would be a member of the first ambulance vehicle at the scene) to a commander of appropriate rank or skilled suitability who has been dispatched specifically to take the role. In protracted incidents, the welfare of incident commanders is as important as that of any other responder. Therefore, there may be the need to establish a Tactical Commander rota. Where this occurs, care must be taken to ensure a complete handover is achieved and documented.

Commanders should interact as shown in Figure 10.5. During major incidents and major incident exercises, it is often the case that communication between Tactical Commanders is poor; the effective management of an incident demands good communication and these commanders *must* arrange to meet at regular intervals. In the early phases of the incident a brief discussion may be required every 20 or 30 minutes.

Key point
Good command and control requires good communication both vertically and horizontally.

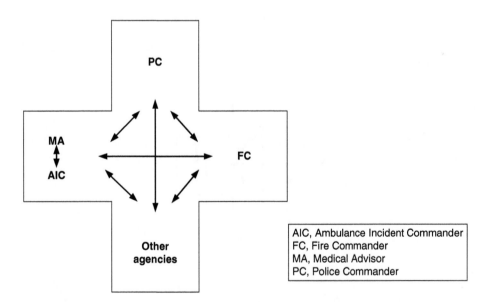

PC

MA

AIC

FC

Other
agencies

AIC, Ambulance Incident Commander
FC, Fire Commander
MA, Medical Advisor
PC, Police Commander

Figure 10.5 The cross of communication

The commanders of each scene may move around to maintain an overview of how the situation is developing but will often concentrate their activity close to the command vehicles. Health service commanders act in leadership roles and therefore must not be involved directly in the rescue process or the treatment of the injured. Their role is to ensure that there are adequate resources at the scene, and that the resources are maintained through resupply of equipment, replacement of personnel and casualty distribution. The organisation of on-scene command is shown in Figure 10.6.

The organisation of the on-scene Operational area is shown in Figure 10.7.

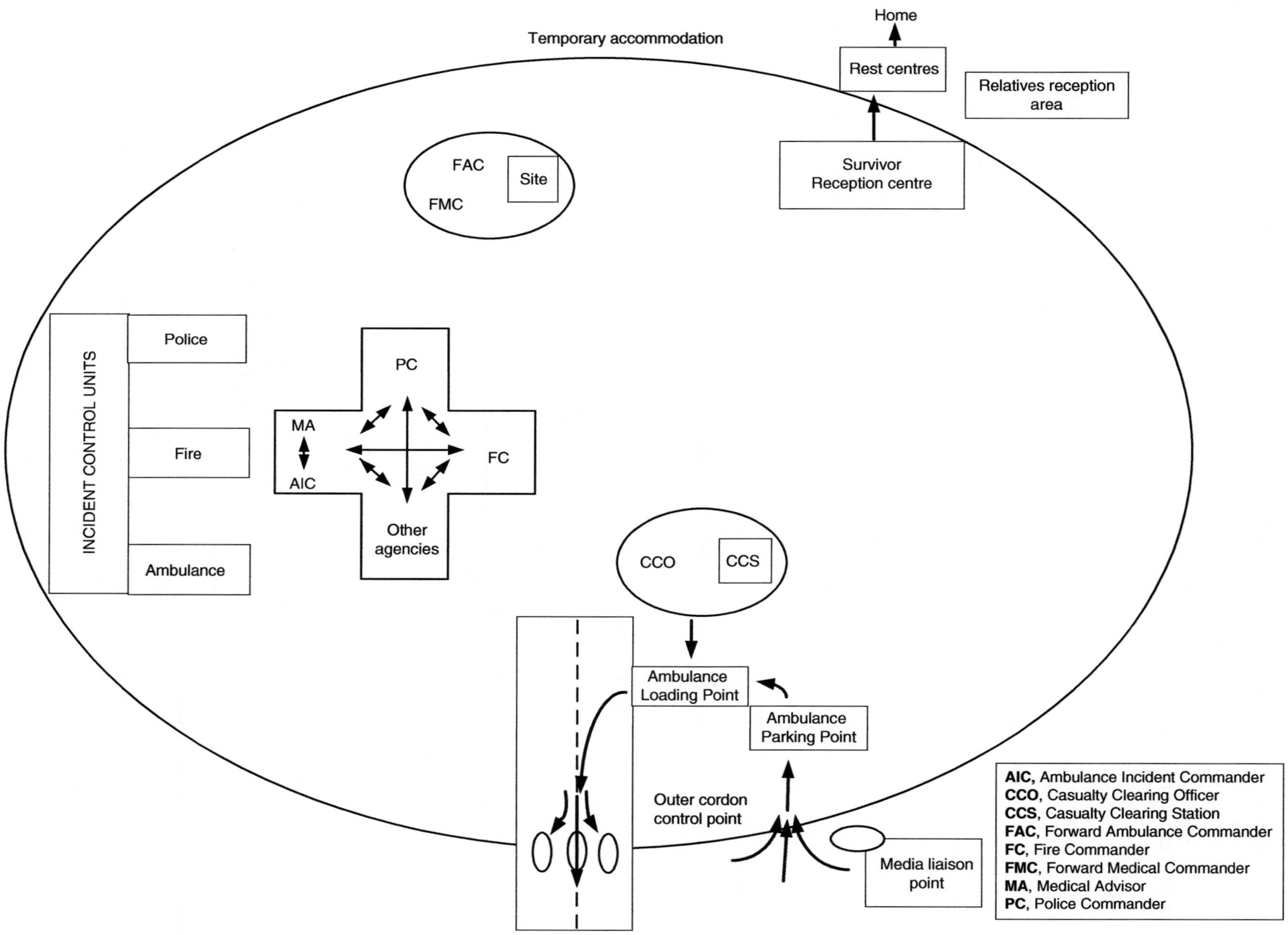

Figure 10.6 On-scene command

AIC, Ambulance Incident Commander
CCO, Casualty Clearing Officer
CCS, Casualty Clearing Station
FAC, Forward Ambulance Commander
FC, Fire Commander
FMC, Forward Medical Commander
MA, Medical Advisor
PC, Police Commander

Relatives reception area

Home

Rest centres

Survivor Reception centre

Temporary accommodation

Media liaison point

Ambulance Parking Point

Ambulance Loading Point

Outer cordon control point

CCS

CCO

Site

FAC

FMC

FC

PC

Other agencies

MA

AIC

Police

Fire

Ambulance

INCIDENT CONTROL UNITS

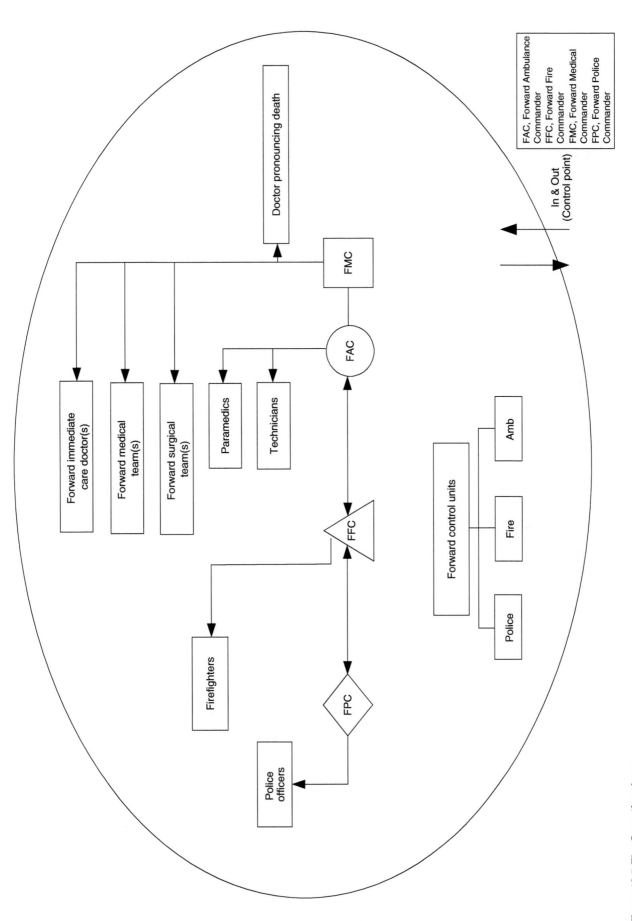

Doctor pronouncing death

FMC

Forward immediate
care doctor(s)

Forward medical
team(s)

Forward surgical
team(s)

Paramedics

Technicians

FAC

FFC

Firefighters

FPC

Police
officers

Forward control units

Police

Fire

Amb

In & Out
(Control point)

FAC, Forward Ambulance
Commander
FFC, Forward Fire
Commander
FMC, Forward Medical
Commander
FPC, Forward Police
Commander

Figure 10.7 The Operational area

Each emergency service has a clearly defined chain of command from their own Tactical Commander through their Operational Commander to individual personnel on the ground. A request for assistance must be passed through this chain to retain command. For example, if a firefighter finds a trapped casualty, they should approach a member of the ambulance service (who will advise the Operational Commander) or the Operational Fire Commander and request support at that location. If requests are not sanctioned through the recognised chain of command, then command is effectively lost and appropriate actions may not occur or may be duplicated.

Key point

Requests for medical assistance at the site must be channeled through commanders. Discipline is required if command is to be maintained.

10.7 Summary

- Each emergency service at the scene has an incident commander
- One service will take overall responsibility for the overall coordination of the management of the incident
- Effective command and control requires good communication between and within services
- There are three tiers of command in relation to a major incident: Operational, Tactical and Strategic. There can be any number of Operational areas within a single incident
- Emergency service command vehicles may co-locate at the scene to form the Joint Emergency Services Control Centre or at a Tactical Coordinating Centre
- Requests for assistance at the scene must pass through the correct chain of command

CHAPTER 11
Health service scene layout

11.1 Introduction

In order to understand how the health service operates at the scene, it is essential to know the way in which it is laid out within the cordons.

11.2 Key locations

Whatever the nature of the incident, it is likely that the health service response will require certain key locations to be established. Figure 11.1 is a schematic representation of these key locations.

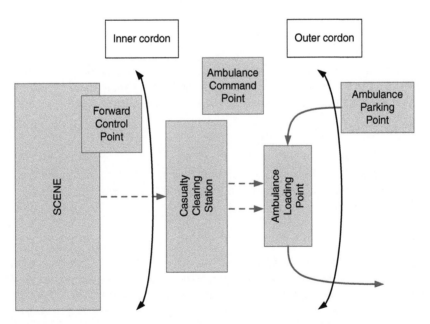

Figure 11.1 Schematic representation of the layout of the health services at a major incident

Major Incident Medical Management and Support: The Practical Approach at the Scene, Fourth Edition.
Edited by Tony Gleeson and Kevin Mackway-Jones.
© 2023 John Wiley & Sons Ltd. Published 2023 by John Wiley & Sons Ltd.

Of course, each incident is different and the exact locations and relationships will vary. It may be necessary to leave some functions out altogether or to duplicate others. For example, if access to particular parts of the scene is difficult, then two Casualty Clearing Stations might be set up, each supported by an Ambulance Loading Point. This will require a greater need for personnel to man the separate Casualty Clearing Stations and Ambulance Loading Points.

Ambulance Command Point

This is the ambulance command vehicle. It may be co-located with other command vehicles at the Joint Emergency Services Control Centre (JESCC).

In the UK, if the predesignated ambulance command vehicle has been deployed, it should be identified with a steady green light. In addition to the green light, standard flashing blue lights may also be used.

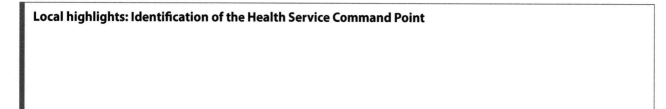

Local highlights: Identification of the Health Service Command Point

The Ambulance Command Point provides a focus for the management of the resources of all the health services, and an on-site communications facility.

> **Key point**
> All health service personnel attending an incident must report to the Ambulance Command Point.

Forward Control Point

This area is close to or within the immediate area of the incident and is selected so that the Operational Commander can direct operations using mobile communications. There may be a need to have more than one Forward Control Point and a number of Operational Commanders to direct different parts of a large scene. These different Operational (Bronze) parts of the scene are known as sectors.

Ambulance Parking Point

This is essentially a holding area where ambulances are kept until they are called forward to the Ambulance Loading Point. Ideally access both from the arrival route and the scene should be good. In prolonged incidents, this area becomes a focus for staff briefing, resupply and refreshment.

Casualty Clearing Station

This area is normally established by the ambulance service and supported by other clinicians. It serves as a focus for secondary triage and the treatment of casualties. The only absolute requirement is that this area should be safe. Access (both from the scene and to evacuation routes), shelter, light and size also need to be considered. The Ambulance Loading Point (see following) is adjacent to it.

> **Key point**
> When the Casualty Clearing Station is established, factors such as safety, access, shelter and size should be considered.

When the Casualty Clearing Station is set up outside, the areas intended for casualties of different priorities should be clearly marked (Figure 11.2). This may be done with different colour (red/yellow/green) groundsheets, separate structures, inflatable tents or simply a stick in the ground with a triage label of the corresponding colour attached. When tents or other structures are used, they should not be crammed with stretcher patients, this simply transfers patients from one entrapment situation (the incident) into another (the tent or structure). Close packing of stretchers not only limits access to the patients but also restricts the flow of casualties through the area. Patients should be placed in the Casualty Clearing Station with their heads towards the centre to allow access to their airway and to allow support of their breathing.

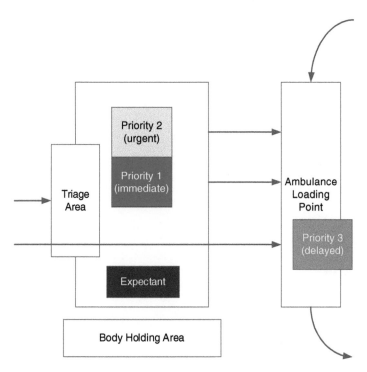

Figure 11.2 Schematic representation of a Casualty Clearing Station

Casualties can be moved between the treatment areas, depending upon whether they improve or deteriorate. A similar flow should be possible within the evacuation area. This system allows for those patients whose priority changes during treatment or while awaiting evacuation.

Ambulance Loading Point

This is the area where ambulances collect casualties from the Casualty Clearing Station for transportation to hospital or other health care facilities. A key role of the Ambulance Loading Officer at this point is to ensure an accurate record of when and where casualties are sent from the scene.

11.3 Control of key areas

One of the most important steps in converting the chaos of a major incident into organised treatment, is to establish control of the flow of patients. Equipment must be available to demarcate key areas and to signpost them. Plastic tape (green check to distinguish it from the blue and red tapes used by the police and fire services, respectively) can be used to control entry and exit points. Collapsible signposts can help to indicate the key clinical areas. The ambulance service commonly has tents (inflatable or other rapid deployment structures) that can provide a sheltered area for holding and treating casualties prior to transport.

Local highlights: Equipment for the control of key areas

11.4 Summary

- The site plan involves establishing an Ambulance Command Point (as part of the Joint Emergency Services Control Centre), Forward Control Point(s), Casualty Clearing Station(s) and Ambulance Loading Point(s)
- In order to establish and maintain the flow of ambulances for evacuation of casualties, a circuit must be set up. An Ambulance Parking Point should be set up first

CHAPTER 12
Safety at the scene

Learning outcomes

After reading this chapter you will be able to:
- Discuss the safety priorities at the scene
- Describe how to safely approach the scene
- Describe the role of the Ambulance Safety Officer
- Define the basic principles of risk assessment at the scene

---

12.1 Introduction

One of the first principles of pre-hospital emergency care is 'do not become a casualty yourself'. A responder to an incident is of little use to anyone if they become a casualty. Responder casualties may in fact make the situation significantly worse as they not only deplete the available pool of resources but also add an additional burden to an already stretched healthcare system.

Every individual has a duty to take reasonable steps to ensure their own safety and to properly use the safety equipment provided. There is no way of guaranteeing absolute safety in an operational incident, but by following a few simple rules and being aware of the environment, the risks can be minimised.

12.2 Health and safety legislation

Most countries have placed an obligation on employers to minimise the risk to their employees from work-related dangers. This legislation usually extends to all but the most severe incidents that emergency services respond to.

Local highlights: Relevant health and safety legislation

12.3 The 1-2-3 of safety

Responders should follow the 1-2-3 of safety. In order of priority:

1. Self safety.
2. Scene safety.
3. Survivor(s) safety.

Major Incident Medical Management and Support: The Practical Approach at the Scene, Fourth Edition.
Edited by Tony Gleeson and Kevin Mackway-Jones.
© 2023 John Wiley & Sons Ltd. Published 2023 by John Wiley & Sons Ltd.

Self safety

A responder's first priority must always be to ensure their personal safety. There may be situations where risk assessments have been carried out for a particular task or area of work. Responders should be familiar with these risk assessments and understand any steps they need to take to minimise risk. In addition, a dynamic risk assessment should be carried out and documented throughout the incident as shown in Figure 12.1.

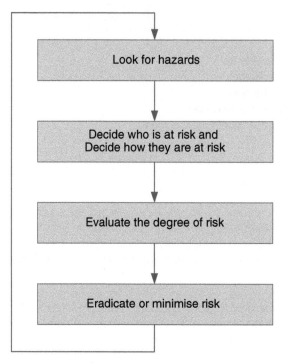

Figure 12.1 Dynamic risk assessment

It is always important to approach with caution – this allows time for risk assessment. Hazardous substances may be the cause of any incident, even if the nature of the call does not suggest it. Responders should maintain an index of suspicion throughout and should always follow the principles shown in Tables 12.1 and 12.2.

Table 12.1 The safe approach

Action	Reason
Approach upwind and uphill of the incident	Minimises exposure to contamination trail
Go to rendevous point if identified	Ensures appropriate reporting and deployment
Stop at first fire appliance (unless closer than 100 m)	May be standing off or have information
Stay a minimum of 100 m from the incident	Minimises risk from explosion
Retreat if continuous loud noise	May indicate leak under pressure
Wear maximum personal protective equipment available	Protects from contaminants
Obtain treatment if contaminated	Early treatment improves outcome

Table 12.2 Safety triggers for emergency personnel (STEP 1-2-3) to assist in identifying the possibility of hazardous materials incidents

Step 1	*One* casualty, incapacitated with no obvious reason	Approach using normal procedures
Step 2	*Two* casualties, incapacitated with no obvious reason	Approach with caution using normal procedures
Step 3	*Three or more* casualties, in close proximity, incapacitated with no obvious reason	DO NOT APPROACH THE SCENE, implement REMOVE, REMOVE, REMOVE procedures

There may also be other signs, which might be useful in confirming the release of a hazardous material, and these are dealt with in more detail in Chapter 19.

Personal protective equipment

Personal protective equipment should be worn if indicated. This is described in detail in Chapter 7.

Scene safety

Ambulance Safety Officer

The Ambulance Safety Officer reports to the Ambulance Incident Commander and is responsible for the overall safety of all health personnel at the site of a major incident. It may be appropriate to deploy a number of safety officers or assistants dependent on the need of the incident. They will ensure that all ambulance and other health service staff wear the correct high-visibility and protective clothing. Together with the other emergency services, specialist advisor(s) and decontamination officer(s) they will identify the risks and hazards present in the area of operation. Finally, they will monitor correct working practices at the scene. These tasks are shown in Box 12.1.

Box 12.1 Ambulance Safety Officer tasks

- Liaise with any other specialist safety advisors present
- Identify any actual or potential hazards and ascertain the correct course of action/control measures required. Notify Ambulance Control and the Ambulance Incident Commander of all hazards to ensure safety information is communicated to all staff
- Ensure that all ambulance and health service personnel arriving and working at the site are correctly identified and wear the appropriate high visibility and protective clothing
- Ensure safe working practices are happening and act immediately to manage any risks to the health and safety of staff
- Conduct an analytical risk assessment at regular intervals, recording the information as required
- Liaise with the Ambulance Parking Point Officer to ensure that all staff arriving at the scene are briefed about actual and potential hazards and are correctly attired prior to proceeding on the site
- Monitor the time responders spend on site and make provision for adequate rest and refreshment facilities at the scene
- Immediately advise staff in the inner/outer cordon areas and Ambulance Control/Ambulance Incident Commander in the event evacuation of the scene is required

---

The Ambulance Safety Officer will be identified by a high-visibility tabard inscribed 'Ambulance Safety Officer'.

Analytical risk assessment process

As well as initial dynamic risk assessments, a more detailed approach may be necessary. This is known as the analytical risk assessment. As things will continuously change during an incident, the Ambulance Safety Officer should constantly review and update the assessment of hazards. This should be done at regular intervals or whenever the risk to ambulance and health service personnel changes.

The analytical risk assessment includes the following elements:

- A formalised assessment of the hazards
- An assessment of existing control measures with additional control measures introduced as appropriate

Emergency evacuation signal

The emergency services should have an agreed method to warn responders within the inner cordon of a safety issue that requires immediate evacuation of the site. The signal is often three blasts on a whistle but could also be:

- The sounding of an air horn/car horn
- A radio message transmitted to all call-signs
- Coded warning

Whichever method is used it must be agreed by the emergency services prior to the deployment of operational personnel. The emergency evacuation signal must be understood by everyone in attendance at the incident scene.

Survivor(s) safety

Survivor safety is an important issue – there is little point in deploying health service staff to save life, only to see lives lost because of failure to identify and manage hazards.

Survivor safety may include:

- Removal to a place of safety away from the incident site, for example:
  - Use of safe buildings for shelter, for example a Survivor Reception Centre
  - Use of ambulance service tented structures
- In the case of a contaminated casualty:
  - The removal of contaminated clothing
  - Assessment of the need for decontamination
- Provision of warm blankets, clothing, etc.

12.4 After the incident is over

During the closing stage of an incident, complacency can set in. The process of task and hazard identification, the assessment of risk and the planning, organisation, control, monitoring and review of the preventive and protective measures must continue until the last resource leaves the incident scene. The Ambulance Commander should have no hesitation in halting work in order to maintain safety.

It is important that systems are in place to monitor the health of staff following an incident. As a matter of course, incident commanders will take advice as to any immediate treatment and monitoring that staff should undergo if they have been exposed to any hazardous substance. Health and safety departments, occupational health services, employee counselling services and peer support networks are valuable sources of advice and support. In addition to this, a written record of individual staff involvement/exposure at an incident should be retained.

12.5 Summary

- Safety is extremely important at the scene of a major incident and may be governed by legislation
- The 1-2-3 of safety should be followed
- A risk assessment should be performed by the first crew arriving at the scene
- The Ambulance Safety Officer should undertake analytical risk assessments regularly during the incident
- Safety monitoring should carry on until the last resource has left the scene
- After the incident is over the health of staff should be monitored as required

CHAPTER 13
Communications

Learning outcomes

After reading this chapter you will be able to:
- Discuss why good communications are important
- Describe methods of communication that can be used at a major incident
- Discuss what is needed to establish a communications structure

---

13.1 Introduction

Good communications are essential for an effective major incident response. Without good communications the emergency services cannot deliver a coordinated response. Poor communication is recurrently identified as a problem when major incident management is investigated.

'I was left with the clear impression that opportunities to pass vital information between the services were missed.'

Desmond Fennell OBE QC, investigation into the King's Cross Underground fire

'Emergency services shall carry out exercises simulating a major incident on a regular basis to test specifically their communication systems in the light of the shortcomings identified . . .'

Anthony Hidden QC, investigation into the Clapham Junction railway accident

'The key to an effective response to a major or catastrophic incident is communication. This includes communication within and between the emergency, health, transport and other services. It also includes effective communication with the individuals caught up in the incident, and the public at large.'

London Assembly Report of the 7 July Review Committee, 2006

Good communication is *complete, accurate and timely*. It is designed to ensure that everyone who needs to know is informed as soon as possible. Systems should be in place to not only show that messages were passed, but also to record that they were received and acted on. To achieve this, good communication must be part of preparation – plans should include it, equipment must be in place and staff who are expected to communicate must be trained to do so.

Major Incident Medical Management and Support: The Practical Approach at the Scene, Fourth Edition.
Edited by Tony Gleeson and Kevin Mackway-Jones.
© 2023 John Wiley & Sons Ltd. Published 2023 by John Wiley & Sons Ltd.

The consequences of bad communication can be severe. If, for example, a shortage of equipment at the Casualty Clearing Station is not communicated, there will be no resupply: this is a *lack of information*. If the sender of the message does not confirm with the receiver that the message is understood, the wrong action may be taken, for example a need for 'Entonox' may become a need for an 'empty box': this is *failure to confirm the information*. If messages are not logged with the Ambulance Service Control Vehicle at the scene, requests may not be actioned or may be carried out in duplicate: this is a *lack of coordination*.

Key point

Good communication is crucial to the effective management of a major incident.

13.2 Communication methods

The following methods of communication will be discussed:

- Radios (airwave terminal or handset)
- Telephones (mobile, land line, internet or satellite)
- Other methods including runners, pagers, loud-hailers, whistles, hand signals, public announcements, television and radio broadcasts and multimedia communication devices

Radios

Before using a radio, it is important to know:

- Who can be contacted: radio net/talkgroups/channels
- How the radio is operated: the working parts/battery, etc.
- The correct form of speech: radio voice procedure

Traditional analogue radio net

On a traditional radio net, each person who uses the radio has an identifying name or number. This is known as a 'call-sign'. Everyone who uses a radio is on an allocated frequency and this is part of a 'radio net'. Each emergency service operates on a separate frequency and therefore has its own radio net. Messages are usually passed from an individual to a control room vehicle. An example of a radio net is shown in Figure 13.1. 'Control' can hear everyone and speak to everyone, but individuals may only be able to hear and speak to the control room vehicle, depending upon the operating system.

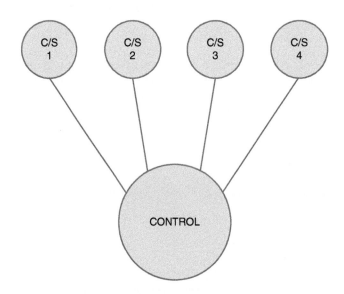

Figure 13.1 A radio net.
C/S, call-sign

Single frequency simplex: All users transmit and receive on the same frequency. All users can therefore be heard by, and can speak to, each other provided each set is powerful enough. This is also referred to as an 'open' channel and is desirable in a major incident so that all key officers can monitor the progress of the incident.

Duplex: Users transmit and receive on separate frequencies. Each user can only talk directly to and can only hear Control (unless Control organises *talk-through*). Control can speak to and hear all stations. This is the usual ambulance service operational system for daily use.

If a user has a hand-held radio as well as a radio in a vehicle, the same call-sign is usually retained (whichever radio set is being used at the time). In a major incident scenario, call-signs for hand-held radios will change, depending on the role of the individual.

Key point

Only one person can transmit on any radio net at any one time.

Radios can operate on HF (high frequency), VHF (very high frequency) or UHF (ultra high frequency). HF radios have the longest range and UHF the shortest. Traditional ambulance service radios have usually been VHF and allow communication with the Health Services Command Vehicle at the scene, with Ambulance Control and directly with the hospital (if they have a receiver installed). UHF radios have often been distributed on the scene for use by key health personnel, but are unlikely to have a range that will allow communication much beyond the scene. HF radios may be utilised in remote areas or by military personnel.

Since the late 1990s, it has become apparent that the old analogue VHF/UHF frequencies that were being used to provide radio communication networks were no longer able to deliver the bandwidth necessary for development. As such there is a move worldwide to use more modern communication methods. Whatever method is being used locally, it is important to ensure familiarity with the system and the radio devices in use.

Digital hand-held terminals

Throughout the UK, the emergency services currently use a digital radio system. Although this is currently being phased out and the system is being moved onto a dedicated part of the 4G/LTE mobile phone network (Emergency Service Network).

The current digital system, as defined by the European Telecommunications Standards Institute, is designed to provide emergency services with a single, cohesive, digital network that will support multiple teams.

Improvements over VHF radio service will include:

- Improved geographical coverage
- Improved voice quality
- Increased capacity
- Reliability and functionality
- Voice and data
- Greater security of information with encryption built in
- Emergency calls enabling an open microphone on the talkgroup
- Multiple talkgroups

The system enables multiple modes of operation that will allow both secure voice calls and data packages to be sent and received using just the one terminal. The forthcoming system enhances the critical data package to support the delivery of all types of media, including access to databases and video transfer.

Modes of operation

1. *Point-to-point*: Individual private calls between two terminals using the network.
2. *Group calls*: Trunk mode operation between terminals on a set talkgroup.

3. *Direct mode:* Individual call between terminals without using the network.
4. *Multiple talk*: The ability to join a selection of pre-programmed talkgroups.
5. *Emergency calls*: A high-priority call that enables an open microphone on the talkgroup.

The ambulance service has overall responsibility for planning, providing and coordinating health service communications at the scene, and to and from the scene of a major incident.

The requirements for health service communications during a major incident are summarised in Box 13.1.

Box 13.1 Requirements for health service communications during a major incident

On site

Equipment to allow radio communication with and between:
- Key ambulance and medical personnel at the incident
- Ambulance vehicles at the scene
- Ambulance Control
- The incident and receiving hospitals
- The police and fire services

Off site

Radio communications with:
- The Ambulance Command Vehicle at the scene
- Ambulance vehicles travelling to the scene or to hospital
- The receiving hospitals
- Neighbouring ambulance services
- Hospital Ambulance Liaison Officer(s)

Communication from the scene to the receiving hospitals may be direct, or indirect via Ambulance Control. The benefit of the indirect approach is that it allows the health service commanders to concentrate on the scene management. Hospitals need to know specific information: how many patients, estimated time of arrival and clinical severity (triage priorities). Clinical details of individual patients are not required for the hospital to activate their major incident plan and respond appropriately.

Radio working parts and radio voice procedure

To use a radio requires knowledge of the working parts: how to turn it on, select the channel and change a battery. This is dealt with in Appendix D. Using a radio also requires knowledge of how to initiate a message and end a message, and the key words of 'radio shorthand'; this is referred to as radio voice procedure and is also explained in Appendix D with worked examples.

Telephones

Mobile phones

The mobile phone has some benefits as a communication tool in pre-hospital care:

- It allows unrestricted conversation and radio voice procedure is unnecessary
- It allows communication with individuals outside the radio net
- It allows direct communication with hospitals
- It has national (and international) coverage

There are, however, disadvantages to the use of mobiles at a major incident:

- There is no central coordination of messages
- There is no centrally recordable audit of conversations
- There are limited cells available, and saturation of the system can rapidly occur

The absence of central coordination of messages will mean that there is no log of important requests – thus requests will not be routinely followed up if they fail to be actioned. Failure of coordination may also lead to a duplication of effort, counter-orders and a breakdown in the control of the health service response scene.

As mobiles do not normally have a recording capability, there is the opportunity for key messages to be missed. Following any major incident there will be a post-incident inquiry that will scrutinise communications between commanders. Failure to record or log these messages may result in criticism regarding areas of responsibility or miscommunication (see Appendix C).

As there are a limited number of cells, they can rapidly become occupied by members of the media, public and survivors. This can be overcome by having a reserved number of cells that can be activated in an emergency and accessed only by emergency service personnel who have modified phones (Mobile Telephone Preference Access Scheme – MTPAS). The modification of mobiles for this purpose requires rigid control. Planning is required to ensure that an incident commander's telephone is protected in this way.

> **Key point**
>
> Messages should be passed through the Ambulance Control Vehicle to maintain control and recording of the health service's response.

Land lines

A field telephone system may be useful to connect fixed points around the incident, for example the Command Vehicle, Forward Control Point and Casualty Clearing Station. Long messages or secure information can be sent over this network rather than the radio. Information cannot be recorded on this system.

In protracted incidents (days), it may be possible for a telecommunications provider to install new land lines.

Within a hospital, the telephone is the principal form of communication. Messages should be kept short and alternative methods of communication, such as runners, should be considered. Additional telephone points may be necessary within areas designated for major incident administration, with the telephones only used when the plan is activated.

A police casualty documentation team will be sent to every receiving hospital to collect information on all patients treated. A central casualty bureau will collate the information from the hospitals together with information from the scene. The media, on instruction from the police, will broadcast a public contact number for the casualty bureau.

A hospital switchboard may become rapidly saturated with calls in a major incident. These may come from staff answering the activation cascade, from the media and from relatives or friends of the injured. It is the responsibility of the hospital's management team to provide a system that will cope with the increase in demand of calls and to regularly test this system.

Other methods

Runners

At the scene, the use of runners should always be considered. They are a reliable method to pass information and often faster than trying to make contact over a very busy radio net. It may be appropriate to send handwritten messages to avoid degradation of the content of the message. Runners must have the appropriate personal protective equipment.

> **Key point**
>
> Runners are reliable and may be faster than using the radio.

Hand signals

Hand signals can be adopted, and are useful for communicating in line of sight but where voice cannot be heard because of distance or background noise. They are used frequently by the military and ambulance service special operations teams.

Whistle

A whistle can be used to good effect to attract attention. However, repeated whistle blasts are often used to indicate imminent danger and the need to evacuate the site. This may preclude the use of a whistle for any other purpose at the scene.

Public announcements

Brief messages passed over a megaphone are an effective means of communication with a group of individuals. A public address system may be used to give information to a crowd when an incident occurs at an organised event. Similarly, the electronic information display boards at sports stadia can have public evacuation procedure notices pre-programmed (remember that spoken messages alone may not communicate with those with hearing impairment).

Television and radio broadcasts

Television increasingly broadcasts real-time information from the incident site to the public. This can be useful to off-site commanders and receiving hospitals who gain a better understanding of the scene. In certain circumstances, broadcasters can be used to the advantage of the health and emergency services. An announcement on local radio can warn and inform the general public about the incident and may include information on public health messages and traffic management diversions. This information would be coordinated through the police.

Video downlink

Police forces throughout the UK have helicopters that can video the scene and surrounding area and send real-time images directly to command rooms. This provides vital scene information that would otherwise not be available.

The emergency services may use drone technology to view specific geographical areas, buildings or hot zones to search for casualties and hazards. This has been proven to provide critical information and reduce potential harm to responders.

Data transmission

The ability to transmit data messages can enhance communication during a major incident. Short message service (SMS) and multimedia messaging service (MMS) texts, email and the use of the internet will allow incident commanders access to vital information when necessary. Data transmission also reduces the pressure on the traditional verbal communication infrastructure.

Telemedicine

Systems that allow real-time remote support for the management of a major incident using an internet link from a remote computer with a modem and telephone have been developed. The use of a satellite telephone could allow remote support from anywhere in the world.

Social media

It is highly likely that social media networks will be relaying information and pictures about any incident before there is any emergency service activity on scene. Emergency services need to make best use of this information as it could provide critical information on scene assessment and likely casualty numbers. Also, responders need to be aware that social media will be used to monitor their activity, therefore providing visual evidence of their management of the incident and casualties.

Emergency services should also consider the use of social media to warn and inform the general public. This has been proven to assist those services and the general public during very demanding periods of activity.

13.3 Summary

- Good communications are crucial to the effective management of a major incident
- Radios are in common use
- Alternative methods of communication can be utilised as appropriate
- The use of mobile phones at the scene is convenient but may contribute to a reduction in control and coordination

CHAPTER 14
Assessment

Learning outcomes

After reading this chapter you will be able to:
- Describe why scene assessment is important
- Detail who carries out the initial scene assessment
- Describe what should be included in the initial scene assessment
- Define what constitutes subsequent scene assessment

14.1 Introduction

The initial and ongoing assessments of the scene are fundamental to both single service and joint service scene management. The initial assessment needs to provide sufficient information not only to allow the assessor to declare a major incident, but also enough information to ensure that the response is to the right place with the right resources and with minimum risk to the rescuers. Subsequent continuous scene assessments will inform the response as it evolves and will ensure that decisions are made with the best available facts. Any risks identified should undergo a dynamic risk assessment and a plan made to eliminate, reduce or mitigate them.

14.2 Initial assessment

As has been noted already, assessment is an integral part of the overall CSCA scene management approach. The initial scene assessment by the health services should be carried out by the first ambulance personnel on the scene – one of whom will become the initial Ambulance Incident Commander. This means that every member of the ambulance crew must be able to carry out an initial scene assessment.

The quality of the first information that is passed from the scene will be important in determining the speed and adequacy of the subsequent response. The acronym METHANE is recommended as a reminder of the key information to be passed.

M	Major incident declaration
E	Exact location
T	Type of incident
H	Hazards
A	Access/egress
N	Number of casualties
E	Emergency services and equipment required

Major Incident Medical Management and Support: The Practical Approach at the Scene, Fourth Edition.
Edited by Tony Gleeson and Kevin Mackway-Jones.
© 2023 John Wiley & Sons Ltd. Published 2023 by John Wiley & Sons Ltd.

Major incident declaration

The Ambulance Communications Officer at the scene will quickly come to realise that the number of live casualties is greater than the resources available to treat them – and that a major incident (in health service terms) has occurred. In large incidents, it may be necessary to estimate rather than give exact numbers of casualties, especially in the early stages of an incident when all information may not be clear. When passing information back to Control, it is important that this fact is communicated clearly at the beginning of the conversation; this will allow the recipient of the information at Control to flag the importance of the message. An early, clear declaration also ensures that there is no element of doubt about expected actions.

Exact location

It is essential that the exact location of the incident is sent immediately. This will help additional resources to arrive as quickly as possible. It can be difficult in some circumstances to be sure exactly where an incident has occurred – and a description of street names, junctions, landmarks and even reference to the crew's vehicle (which should be locatable via the automatic vehicle location system) may help control pinpoint the location precisely.

Type of incident

A general description of the type of incident not only helps control and responders to envisage the scene, but also allows certain predetermined actions to occur. For example, a gas explosion in a block of flats will trigger a different immediate response from the fire service than a multiple vehicle incident. Similarly, the health service immediate response to an aircraft accident will be very different to that for a hazardous materials release.

Hazards

There are likely to be numerous hazards at any major incident scene and it is not reasonable to expect that the initial scene assessment will include a comprehensive hazard risk review. However, a general description of hazard types – such as 'falling masonry' or 'fire' – can be helpful, and specific information about hazardous materials can reduce the risks to rescuers by allowing provision of appropriate personal protective equipment. It is very likely that the sophistication of the hazard report will increase as the incident progresses, so time should not be wasted initially in trying to cover everything.

Access/egress

Again, it is unlikely that there will be time to undertake a full review of routes in and out of a recently occurred major incident. Future responders will benefit from a general description of what can reasonably be found out immediately. For instance, the fact that traffic on a motorway is stationary behind an incident may allow control to plan (with the police) a different approach. Similarly, knowledge about flooded roads or broken bridges can save significant time for later responders.

Number of casualties

Everyone always wants to know the number of casualties involved; this is a key factor in planning the response by the health service. It can be one of the most difficult facts to establish early on in the incident as access to the casualties is usually poor, rumours (usually incorrect) are rife and injuries are hidden. No more than a reasonable estimate is expected as part of an initial assessment – this is best obtained by a rapid, safe scene reconnaissance.

Emergency services and equipment required

Although it is likely that other emergency services will already be attending, it is important to reinforce the need for support from appropriate services via Health Service Control. At this stage, any obvious equipment needs (beyond the usual major incident response) should also be highlighted so that early arrangements can be made. At this point in the assessment, clarity should be provided on the initial number of ambulance resources required at the scene of the incident. This should be in terms of provision of transport and specialist ambulance service resources.

14.3 Continued assessment

Once the initial assessment has been undertaken and has been communicated to Control (using the METHANE report), the Ambulance Incident Commander should continue to refine and update the assessment of the scene from a health service perspective. As further resources arrive and it becomes possible to establish a command and control structure, the Ambulance Incident Commander needs to ensure that subordinate commanders are briefed to feed continual updates from their areas of control. In addition, the Ambulance Incident Commander should continually liaise with other service commanders to glean health-related information.

The continuous assessment process can be structured around the second part of the initial assessment, as shown:

H	Hazards
A	Access/egress
N	Number of casualties
E	Equipment and staff required

This can be used by commanders at all levels.

Hazards

Hazard information continues to be very important, both for decision making and also for planning. Subordinate commanders should ensure that the Ambulance Incident Commander is kept up to date with developing hazards in their areas – often this information will be collated by the Ambulance Safety Officer who will also liaise with other emergency service safety officers and will brief the Ambulance Incident Commander accordingly. When hazards/risks are identified, there are a number of ways of dealing with them: eliminate the hazard (if possible), reduce it, isolate the hazard, put in controls (safe systems of work), use of appropriate PPE and, finally, discipline to avoid (for example by putting appropriate signage).

Access

The routes into and out of the scene will usually be under the control of the police. However, the location of any ambulance and health service rendezvous points and the exact circuit to be used by ambulances within the outer cordon are within the control of the Ambulance Parking Point Officer. Changes in arrangements (perhaps dictated by evolving hazards) form part of continuous scene assessment. Forward Commanders may also report special access routes within the incident site.

Number of casualties

While clarity about the number of casualties involved in the incident does develop with time, collating the information can become increasingly difficult as the scene becomes dynamic. It is essential, therefore, that this aspect of scene assessment is actively managed. Regular reports on the number and nature of casualties (usually expressed in terms of their triage priorities) should be sought from all parts of the scene. Forward Commanders and the Casualty Clearing Officer will be expected to maintain a good understanding of the casualty states in their areas and must feed this information regularly to the Ambulance Incident Commander. This will either be on an ad hoc basis as the Ambulance Incident Commander moves around the scene or using a more formal (usually timed) reporting format. Knowing the total number and the remaining number of casualties at a scene is a basic requirement for appropriate scene management and is also very important in planning the need for hospital resources.

Equipment and staff required

The equipment in an established scene will ideally be managed though an Equipment Officer who will be responsible both for resupply and for identification of extraordinary equipment requirements. Subordinate commanders will need to ensure that their scene assessments include equipment requirements so that the Equipment Officer can arrange for appropriate provision. Initial equipment will come from responding ambulances until the major incident equipment vehicle arrives on scene.

Staff requirements will reflect the number and nature of the casualties at the scene. In some circumstances, specialist medical teams will be needed for particular patients, whilst in prolonged incidents the need is not for specialists but rather for enough staff to ensure proper rest and recuperation. The Ambulance Incident Commander will rely on subordinate commanders to pass this information up in their regular scene assessment reports.

14.4 Responsibility

Scene assessment is the responsibility of all health service commanders – each should continuously assess their area of responsibility using the HANE (from METHANE) format. The information gained should be used both to manage the immediate area and should also be passed up the chain of command to better inform the overall picture.

14.5 Summary

- Scene assessment is essential for both the initiation and evolution of the response to the incident
- The METHANE message gives a structure for initial scene assessment
- Subsequent assessment can be structured as HANE
- This assessment can and should be used continuously by commanders at all levels

PART V
Medical support

CHAPTER 15
Triage

Learning outcomes

After reading this chapter you will be able to:
- Describe what triage is
- Describe when triage is carried out
- Discuss where triage is carried out
- List the priorities that should be used
- Detail how priorities are assigned
- Describe what patient labels should be applied

15.1 Introduction

In a major incident the aim of the emergency services is to provide the best possible care for the greatest number of patients. However, in the early phase of the response, it is unlikely that there will be sufficient numbers of trained staff to deal with all of the patients at the same time. If the best care is to be given to the greatest number of patients, then a method of assigning priorities is necessary. In order to achieve this goal both the severity of the condition of each patient and their relative priority needs to be assessed. This method of assigning priorities is termed triage.

Whenever the number of patients exceeds the available resources, triage will be necessary. Triage is therefore an essential part of major incident planning and preparation. However, not all major incidents will require formal triage to take place. A collapsed building, from which patients may be removed one at a time, is an example of a major incident at which pre-hospital triage may be unnecessary as the capacity (of the health services) will accommodate the load (rate of patients). This differs from incidents such as train crashes where many patients may require simultaneous assessment.

Triage, meaning to sieve or to sort, is the first step in providing medical support at major incidents (Box 15.1).

Box 15.1 The hierarchy of medical support

- **T**riage
- **T**reatment
- **T**ransport

Triage was first described in modern times by Baron Dominique Jean Larrey who was Napoleon's Surgeon Marshal. He introduced a system of sorting the patients who presented to field dressing stations. His aims were military focused rather than medical and the highest priority was given to soldiers who had minor wounds and who could therefore be returned quickly to the battle with minimum treatment. There is no English language record of the use of triage until the First World War. The official history of the US Army in this conflict uses the word 'triage' when describing the physical area where sorting was done, rather than a description of the sorting itself. Triage has developed since then to be the cornerstone of military medicine. In more recent times, it has become a daily management tool within civilian emergency departments.

Major Incident Medical Management and Support: The Practical Approach at the Scene, Fourth Edition.
Edited by Tony Gleeson and Kevin Mackway-Jones.
© 2023 John Wiley & Sons Ltd. Published 2023 by John Wiley & Sons Ltd.

15.2 Aims

The aim of triage, wherever it is done, is not only to deliver the right patient to the right place at the right time but also to 'do the most for the most'. It can be deduced from this that triage principles should be applied whenever the needs of the patients exceed the capacity of the skilled help immediately available.

> **Key point**
>
> Triage principles should be used when either the number of, or the needs of, patients exceed the capacity of the skilled rescuers available.

Thus triage should take place during the management of emergencies ranging from road traffic collisions (where there might be four or five patients and only one or two paramedics in attendance) to major incidents where, despite large numbers of medical, nursing and paramedical staff, the number of patients may be so large that decisions about the order of their care need to be taken to ensure the best overall outcome.

15.3 Timing

Triage is a dynamic rather than a static process. The state of the patient may change for the better or worse either because of a progression of the injuries or due to interventions that are made.

> **Key point**
>
> Triage is a dynamic (continuous) process.

Triage must therefore be repeated many times during the care of a patient. For example, a typical patient might be triaged when first seen, prior to movement from the immediate scene; in the Casualty Clearing Station (CCS), prior to evacuation; on reception in hospital; during resuscitation and treatment; and, if applicable, prior to surgery. In addition to these occasions (that correspond to events external to the patient), a reassessment of priority will be necessary whenever the patient's condition is noted to have changed.

15.4 Site

The primary triage decision (using the modified triage sieve) is likely to be made at the place where the patient is found. A secondary triage decision (using the triage sort) is usually made when the patient arrives at the CCS. However, as triage is a dynamic process, the patient can be re-triaged at any stage if they deteriorate, so a patient may have multiple triage decisions during their patient journey. The choice of triage method used (modified triage sieve or triage sort) will depend on the numbers of patients to be triaged and the available staff to do it. The modified triage sieve is much quicker than the triage sort so if a patient deteriorates, it will usually be repeated as necessary, before arrival at the CCS.

Triage at the scene and on arrival at the CCS are generally regarded as two fixed points in the triage process and are shown in the schematic triage and evacuation map (Figure 15.1). In this scheme it is envisaged that the initial triage (modified triage sieve) at the site will be carried out predominantly by ambulance personnel, while triage at the CCS (triage sort) will often be carried out by more experienced medically trained professions from a variety of backgrounds (ambulance service, pre-hospital care, emergency medicine, etc.). Some patients, particularly those with minor injuries, may be taken in the short term to a 'place of safety' where they should be assessed to confirm that they do not need further health service input. When appropriate transport is available, they may then be taken to a Survivor Reception Centre (if, following assessment, they are confirmed to be uninjured) or to a hospital P3 area for treatment.

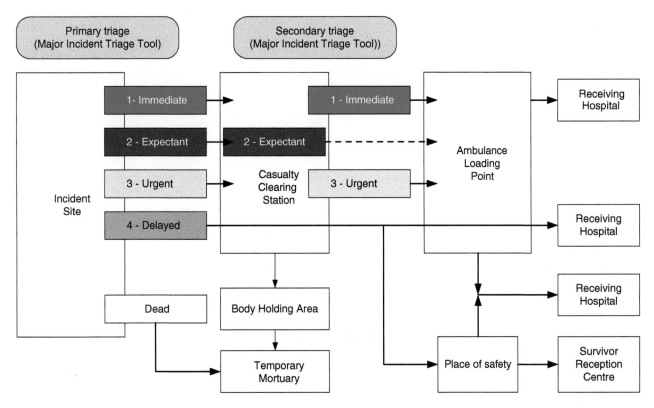

Figure 15.1 Triage and evacuation map

15.5 Priorities

There are four priority systems that are widely used. Two of these are derived from the military, although they are also incorporated into civilian triage labels: they are the 'P' (priority) and the 'T' (treatment) system. Civilian systems are descriptive and colour coded.

The 'P' (priority) system is generally applied to the primary triage process (modified triage sieve) whereas the 'T' (treatment) system is applied to the secondary triage (triage sort) process. All these are summarised in Table 15.1.

Priority system	Treatment System	Category	Colour	Description
Table 15.1 Triage priorities				
P1	T1	Immediate	Red	Patients who require immediate life-saving treatment
P2	T2	Urgent	Yellow	Patients who require surgical or medical intervention within 2–4 hours
P3	T3	Delayed	Green	Less serious cases whose treatment can safely be delayed beyond 4 hours
P4	T4	Expectant	Blue (not standard)	Patients who: Cannot survive treatment Require such a degree of intervention that in the circumstances their treatment would seriously compromise the provision of treatment for others
Dead	Dead	Dead	White or black	Dead

Local highlights: Triage priority

The allocated category in either of the 'P' or 'T' systems reflects the time in which that patient needs to receive treatment, for example:

- *T1, immediate priority*: patients who require immediate life-saving procedures
- *T2, urgent priority*: patients who require surgical or medical intervention within 2–4 hours
- *T3, delayed priority*: less serious cases whose treatment can safely be delayed beyond 4 hours
- *T4, expectant priority*: patients whose condition is so severe that they cannot survive despite the best available care and whose treatment would divert medical resources from salvageable patients who may then be compromised

In a civilian setting the expectant priority will very rarely be activated and generally only if the incident is 'uncompensated' at some point. This is more likely in a natural incident rather than a man-made incident. However, in a military operational setting it is easier to envisage where the tactical situation prevents adequate medical resources being deployed to the scene. The decision to invoke the expectant category will rest jointly with the Health Service Commanders at the scene and may be revoked if adequate resources become available. At this time, any surviving 'expectant' patients will become 'T1, immediate'. The avoidance of the use of this category is probably a mistake, since failure to use it correctly will, on balance, cost lives rather than save them.

It is recognised that some of the available triage labels do not include an independent expectant category. In these circumstances the delayed category can be used, endorsed with 'expectant'. Clearly, these patients must be separated from those with genuine minor injuries.

Key point

Avoiding the use of the expectant category may cost lives.

Local highlights: Rules for invoking the expectant category

15.6 Triage systems

It is essential that all the healthcare providers attending a major incident use the same triage system and the same method for categorising patients into these groups. Historically, different organisations have used different triage priority systems and methods. The confusion that this has caused at the scene and the receiving hospitals is avoidable.

A number of different methods of triage exist worldwide. They are usually based on physiological or anatomical factors or a combination of both. They include:

- Triage sieve
- Modified Physiological Triage Tool 24 (MPTT-24)

- Triage sort (based on the Trauma Revised Triage Score, TRTS)
- START (Simple Triage and Rapid Transport)
- JumpSTART (paediatric version of START)
- SALT (Sort, Assess, Life-saving interventions, Treatment and/or Transport), used in the USA
- CareFlight, used in Australia
- NHS Major Incident Triage Tool (based on the MPTT-24) to be introduced in the UK

Key point

Whichever method is used, it is essential that it is consistently well performed by clinicians across the healthcare system that it is being used in.

The nature of major incidents makes validating these major incident triage tools difficult. The primary triage sieve and the secondary triage sort have been used for many years. However, there is very limited evidence based around the use of the triage sieve. By contrast, the Modified Physiological Triage Tool 24 (MPTT-24) developed by Vassallo et al. (2018), has been found to have the greatest ability of existing triage tools (in civilian and military studies) to identify patients in need of life-saving interventions. The MPTT-24 is very similar to the original triage sieve but incorporates modified physiological values and an assessment of catastrophic haemorrhage (Figure 15.2). As a result of this, there has been a move away from the original triage sieve model to a 'modified triage sieve' based on the physiological values derived from these studies.

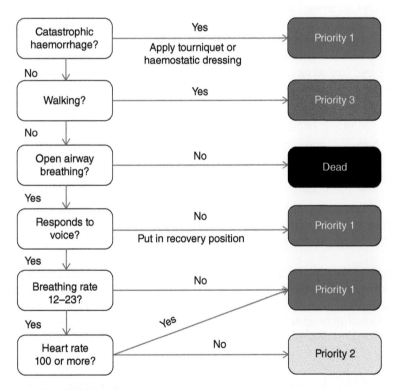

Figure 15.2 The Modified Triage Sieve (MPTT-24).
Source: Vassallo J et al. 2017. Vassallo, J / CC BY 4.0

15.7 Triage methods

Having established the triage categories, it is necessary to provide a reliable method of triage so that all users will come to the same triage decision. There may be considerable numbers of patients and a corresponding number of critical decisions have to be made very quickly. The 'first look' or primary triage (that is carried out by the first rescuers on the scene as a quick assessment of the patients) therefore needs to be rapid, simple, safe and reproducible, irrespective of the background of the provider performing the triage. The modified triage sieve is the rapid triage process that is employed to achieve this.

Key point

Initial triage decisions need to be made quickly, safely and reproducibly irrespective of the provider performing the triage assessment.

Once primary triage has been carried out, more time and resources may be available at the CCS for a more detailed 'secondary triage' assessment. This is the triage sort based on the TRTS. In a situation where there are overwhelming numbers of patients there may never be enough resources for a detailed assessment to take place; in this case either the modified triage sieve or the use of experienced clinician judgement to triage alone will be used for repeated assessments.

Physiological versus anatomical methods

Traditional triage involved 'eye balling' the patient and making a decision based on what injuries could be seen coupled with gut instinct. Such anatomical triage has considerable limitations (Box 15.2). Physiological triage provides an appreciation of the patient's current acuity and relies on detecting changes in vital signs as a result of injury or illness; these systems are more objective, can be performed rapidly without the need to widely expose the patient and require very little training or clinical experience.

Box 15.2 Limitations of anatomical triage

- Patients have to be undressed to see injuries: this is time consuming and impractical
- Decisions are not reproducible between observers with different experience
- Life-threatening injuries may not be detected by examination alone (for example, less than 50% of cases of acute haemoperitoneum are detected by abdominal physical examination alone)
- Exposing patients will lead to a reduction in core body temperature thereby potentially exacerbating any trauma coagulopathy (if present)

Work carried out for the US Navy has shown that non-expert staff can reliably trauma score patients after a very short period of training. The use of such a system is therefore feasible. Furthermore, many modern patient labels (see Section 15.8) incorporate trauma scoring as part of the patient report.

Physiological methods are advantageous as they are quick and reproducible, furthermore they reflect the patient's existing level of acuity. However, they do not take into account the nature of the injury and therefore cannot be used to decide whether a patient should be dispatched to a specialist or a general facility.

By combining anatomical and physiological triage methods discussed earlier, something close to the ideal can be achieved. The rapidity and simplicity of a physiological method such as the triage sort are used to define the initial priority. This can then be supplemented by as much relevant anatomical information as can be obtained in the time and conditions. Thus patients with head injuries can be selected for neurosurgical centres and patients with burns can be sent to regional burns centres, for example. If evacuation is delayed, then anatomical information can be expanded up to the level of a full secondary survey as time allows.

The recommended method of assigning priorities is that the first look triage assessment is carried out at the site of injury using the modified triage sieve. This is followed (usually in the CCS) by a mixed approach to triage using the triage sort to assign priority, supplemented by relevant anatomical information to determine destination.

Key point

- Physiological methods of triage should be used first. These can be supplemented by as much anatomical information as time and conditions allow.

Modified triage sieve

As already stated, this is a physiological-based method of triage. This first look triage quickly sorts the patients into priorities. As it is quick it is not perfect, but any misclassification made at this stage can be corrected later on.

Step 1: Catastrophic haemorrhage

A 'quick look' will assess firstly if there is any evidence of external catastrophic haemorrhage. If there is, then this should be controlled using a tourniquet or haemostatic dressing.

Step 2: Mobility

Patients who can still walk are categorised *P3, delayed*. This is the mobility sieve.

Whilst it is possible to be able to walk with a traumatic upper limb amputation or extensive burns, eventually such patients will collapse and, because the triage process is a dynamic one, they will be reassessed, and their priority will be changed. Remember, the modified triage sieve only provides an assessment of the patient's current physiology following injury, thereby giving a snapshot of their current acuity and not a predictor of what might develop later. Where triage categories are upgraded because of a concern about potential deterioration there will be a disproportionate number of P1 and P2 patients to manage and this can overwhelm limited healthcare resources. This is why triage must be dynamic.

Key point

Walking patients are initially categorised as *P3, delayed* priority.

Step 3: Airway/breathing

Those patients who are not walking are then assessed according to airway, breathing and circulatory (ABC) parameters. If the patient is not breathing, the airway should be opened with a simple manual manoeuvre (head tilt and chin lift or jaw thrust if cervical trauma is suspected) and then reassessed to see if breathing has started. Adult patients who do not breathe despite an airway opening manoeuvre are dead.

If breathing starts when the airway is opened there is an airway problem: these patients are *P1, immediate*. It is clear that an intervention is needed in these patients as they may stop breathing when the airway manoeuvre is released. A bystander can be used to maintain the airway position, a simple airway adjunct can be inserted or the patient quickly turned into the recovery position. It is appropriate for anyone undertaking primary triage to carry both simple airway adjuncts and appropriate dressings or tourniquets in order to control potential catastrophic haemorrhage in patients who may be bleeding.

Key point

Adult patients who cannot breathe despite simple airway manoeuvres are dead.

Step 4: Conscious level assessment

An assessment of the patient's conscious level should now be undertaken using the AVPU (Alert, responds to Voice, responds to Pain, Unconscious) score. If the patient does not respond to voice at this stage, they should be put into the recovery position, have an airway adjunct inserted and/or have bystander help and categorised as *P1, immediate*.

Step 5: Respiratory assessment

For those patients who are responding to voice at this stage, a breathing assessment is then made. Respiratory rate is used as an objective assessment of adequacy, with rates of 12–23 breaths per minute regarded as normal in this situation. A low (less than 12 breaths/min) or high (greater than or equal to 24 breaths/min) respiratory rate indicates a breathing problem: these patients are *P1, immediate*.

Key point

Patients with respiratory rates of 24 or above, or below 12, breaths per minute are *P1, immediate* priority.

Step 6: Circulation assessment

If the rate is normal (between 12 and 23 breaths/min), an assessment of the 'circulation' is made, although this can be difficult in the pre-hospital environment. The pulse rate is checked and those patients with a rate of 100 or more per minute will be *P1, immediate*. A capillary refill assessment may be used instead, with a capillary refill of greater than 2 being abnormal and making the patient a *P1, immediate*. Capillary refill is much less reliable than pulse so a pulse rate is preferred. If the pulse is less than 100 or (if used) capillary refill is 2 seconds or less, then the patient is assigned to *P2, urgent*.

Key point

Patients with a pulse rate of 100 or more beats per minute are *P1, immediate* priority.

Key point

Not all the steps have to be followed. Once a triage decision has been established, further steps do not need to be done. For example, if the patient is mobile their triage decision is P3 and you are not required to do the other steps.

Local learning: Coroner's inquest into London bombings, 7 July 2005

The recommendation following the Coroner's inquest into the 2005 London bombings was that triage training should be reviewed such that immediate medical interventions could be provided (limited to simple airway opening maneouvres and the control of catastrophic haemorrhage) alongside the triage process. Subsequently, the London Ambulance Service has designated 'triage teams', where one provider conducts the triage whilst the other performs immediate life-saving interventions as required.

Paediatric triage tape

The physiological parameters for the modified triage sieve are based on adult ranges. Should these be applied to small children there will be an artificially high triage priority assigned. Some think this is desirable as children should be removed from the incident site as quickly as possible. However, paediatric assessment and treatment resources are generally limited and if these are overstretched further at the hospital level because of over-triage there may be insufficient capacity to deal with the genuine high-priority cases. For this reason, a specific method of paediatric triage has traditionally been considered to be beneficial.

The paediatric triage tape uses the concept that between the ages of 1 and 10 years, length is directly proportional to age, weight and vital signs (Figure 15.3). From this, a series of triage sieve algorithms have been produced using the best available

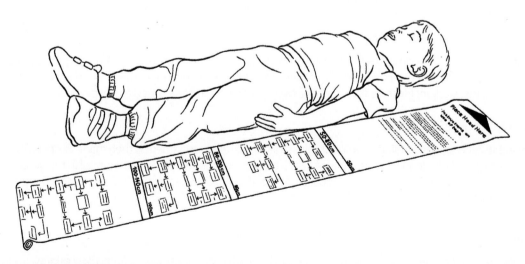

Figure 15.3 Paediatric triage tape.
Reproduced with permission of TSG Associates LLP

guidelines for normal ranges of vital signs. These algorithms are arranged in boxes on a linear waterproof tape that is laid next to the child. The appropriate algorithm is the one next to the child's heel, as illustrated in Figure 15.3. The adult triage sieve is changed in a number of ways. Firstly, very small children cannot walk and therefore the mobility component of the sieve is altered accordingly. Secondly, the value of capillary refill is also questionable and it is only used to screen out abnormalities: in other words, if it is normal the child is *P2, urgent* but an abnormal value still requires a pulse to be taken. Finally, the importance of bradycardia in critical hypovolaemia is recognised and lower limits of pulse rate are given. If the child is trapped a *P1, immediate* priority is assigned until the child is released when objective re-triage can be performed. The modified triage sieve does not support the allocation of *P4, expectant* in either adults or children as it is too quick an assessment to do this accurately.

Local highlights: Paediatric triage

Triage sort

Once patients arrive in the CCS they can be re-triaged in a more controlled manner, providing that there are resources available to allow this. This secondary triage process is typically performed using the triage sort, which comes from the Triage Revised Trauma Score (TRTS).

In previous studies, the TRTS has been shown to be highly sensitive for predicting mortality (in excess of 95%). The TRTS is based on just three physiological parameters: respiratory rate, systolic blood pressure and Glasgow Coma Scale (GCS) score. These parameters are coded as shown in Table 15.2 to give a score from 0 to 12. The triage sort includes an additional step to the TRTS which is the ability to upgrade a patient's priority following a review from a senior clinician.

Table 15.2 Triage Revised Trauma Score system

Physiological variable	Measured value	Score
Respiratory rate (breaths/min)	10–29	4
	>29	3
	6–9	2
	1–5	1
	0	0
Systolic blood pressure (mmHg)	≥90	4
	76–89	3
	50–75	2
	1–49	1
	0	0
Glasgow Coma Scale score	13–15	4
	9–12	3
	6–8	2
	4–5	1
	3	0

The TRTS can be used to assign triage priorities as shown in Figure 15.4 and Table 15.3.

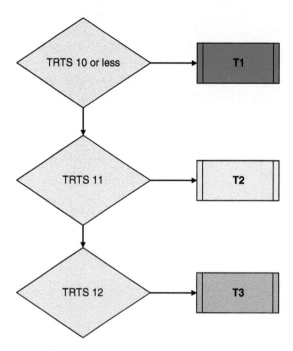

Figure 15.4 Triage Revised Trauma Score

Table 15.3 Triage priorities using the TRTS score in the triage sort	
Treatment	**TRTS score**
T1	1–10
T2	11
T3	12
Dead	0

15.8 Triage labelling

There is little point in triaging patients into priorities if other rescuers are not made aware of the results of the assessment. Some form of labelling is necessary.

To be maximally effective a triage label should be highly visible, should use the standard categories (numbers, words and colours) discussed previously and should be easily and firmly secured to the patient. The label must also allow the patient's priority to be altered as their condition changes.

> **Key point**
>
> Triage labels must be highly visible, easily and securely attached and allow for priorities to be changed.

It is helpful if triage labels themselves can be used for making other clinical notes in the field. In general, the primary colours are preferred since these show up better under difficult ambient lighting conditions. The labelling of the dead is important; the dead label can either be part of the standard triage label or may be a special card designed for this purpose.

Types of label

In broad terms, two types of triage label exist: single and folding.

Single card

When using single cards, a label marked with the appropriate priority is attached to the patient; labels generally consist of a piece of coloured card with printed headings and space for patient information. The single label system is illustrated in Figure 15.5. Since a single coloured card is attached to the patient, changing between categories is relatively difficult as the first card must be removed prior to the new card being attached. This is doubly disadvantageous if notes about the patient have been made on the first card since either this card must be left in place or the notes that have been made on it must be transferred to the new card. If the first card is left then confusion can arise about the current category of the patient.

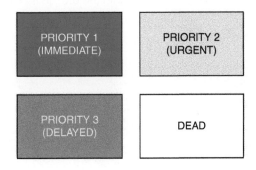

Figure 15.5 Single label system

In general, single label cards are a poor tool if dynamic triage is to be carried out.

> **Key point**
>
> Single card triage labelling systems are not ideal for dynamic triage.

A variation on the single label card is the *Mettag* label (Figure 15.6). This consists of a label that has a number of colour-coded perforated strips on its bottom edge; each strip accords to a different triage category. The strips that do not apply to the

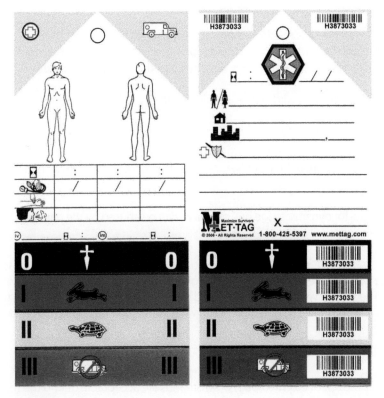

Figure 15.6 Mettag MT137 triage label.
Reproduced with permission of the American Civil Defense Association

patient are removed by the rescuer performing triage and the lowest strip remaining therefore corresponds to the patient's priority. This card has two disadvantages. First, if the patient gets better then it is necessary either to replace the card or to stick the strips that have been torn off back on (i.e. the patient can only deteriorate dynamically). Second, the strip on the card designating the priority is not large and is therefore not visible from a distance. This makes it difficult for a triage officer or another rescuer to look around and assess the number of patients in a particular category in a particular area.

Folding card

The second general approach is the use of a folding card and, within the UK, this is what is most frequently used, with a large number of ambulance trusts using the SMART triage tag (Figure 15.7).

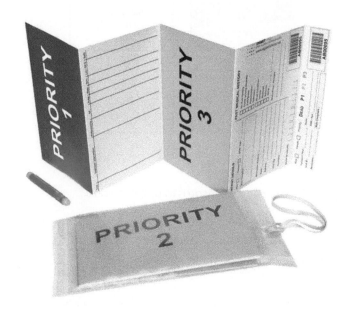

Figure 15.7 SMART tag.
Reproduced with permission of TSG Associates LLP

The cards are folded in such a way that only the desired one of the four priorities is left on the outside; if the priority is changed then it is a simple matter to refold the card and show the new priority on the outside. This system overcomes the problem of additional data since the same card can be used however many times the priority is changed.

Other potential dynamic solutions include card sets and laminated folding card strips.

Key point

Folding triage labels can be used from the time of first triage on the scene to final triage in the receiving hospital.

These cards are extremely useful for dynamic triage but, of course, can be abused by the patients themselves who may refold them to give themselves a higher priority.

Although triage labelling is essential, it is not always necessary to use the complex triage cards discussed earlier. Coloured pegs corresponding to the triage category are quite adequate during the first look triage (triage sieve) and are easily carried on the belt of a rescuer's clothing. The 'slap on wristband', colour coded in the same way, allows the person triaging to quickly identify each category by attaching an appropriate coloured band to a wrist rather than having to fold a label to the correct status.

Key point

Simple alternatives such as the use of coloured pegs or wristbands are acceptable during the triage sieve.

Local highlights: Triage labels in use

15.9 Personnel

Triage is an essential but difficult task. It should always be carried out by trained staff. Over the course of an incident, the person triaging may change from an ambulance paramedic to a senior clinician. Whoever does it, the principles are the same.

15.10 The NHS Major Incident Triage Tool (MITT)

Within the UK there has been a move away from the traditional sieve and sort models to a single, modified triage system, known as the NHS Major Incident Triage Tool (MITT) (Figure 15.8) which is based on the MPTT-24. This is being introduced in autumn 2022 and will be used for adults and children alike for all major incidents in the UK.

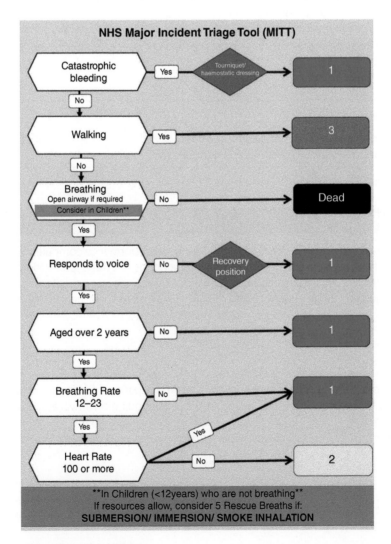

Figure 15.8 The NHS Major Incident Triage Tool (MITT)
Source: Modified from Vassallo J, Cowburn P, Moran CG, Smith JE. The new NHS Prehospital Major Incident Triage Tool: from MIMMS to MITT. *Emerg Med J* 2022.

The new triage tool has been developed from the work done by Vassallo et al. (2018) and was further adapted to include paediatric patients. The MITT is very similar to the modified triage sieve discussed earlier in this chapter, with the same normal physiological values for respiratory rate (rate 12–23 breaths/min) and pulse rate (99 or less per minute) and the assessment of conscious level using the AVPU scale.

With studies demonstrating that the modified triage sieve (MPTT-24) outperformed existing paediatric major incident triage tools (including the paediatric triage tape) in identifying patients in need of life-saving intervention, the MITT has been adapted so that it can also be used with children, thereby allowing a single triage process for both adults and children. It will have a tendency to over-triage children, especially the younger ones, as their normal physiological values differ considerably from adults. This over-triage may be beneficial, in that it removes younger children, who are known to deteriorate rapidly after a period of compensation, sooner from the scene. However, this may have the potential to be problematic if the incident involves a large number of children and in this case, a senior clinician should use their clinical acumen, in association with the MITT, to decide on treatment and transport priorities.

Furthermore, the MITT includes two additional paediatric-specific elements. Firstly, owing to the increased mortality and need for life-saving interventions in the under 2 cohort, all children under 2 years who are not dead are automatically categorised as the highest priority. Secondly, in children under 12 years who are not breathing on opening the airway, and where adequate resources are available, the MITT allows for 5 rescue breaths to be performed where the cause of injury is submersion/immersion or smoke inhalation injuries. Those who respond to 5 rescue breaths are subsequently categorised as the highest priority; they may require an airway adjunct or further breathing support. The triage clinician should be careful not to get task focused on respiratory support of these children and should hand over to a bystander or another clinician and continue the triage process. In a major incident situation, if simple manoeuvres do not work, the primary triage process takes precedence over the treatment of a single patient. Good practice is that the triage process is undertaken in pairs (where numbers of responders allow).

> **Key point**
>
> In children under 12 years of age who are not breathing, if they are victims of immersion, submersion or smoke inhalation and *if resources allow*, consider 5 rescue breaths when using the NHS MITT.

Secondary triage (UK practice)

With evidence demonstrating that the TRTS/triage sort has reduced performance compared with the modified triage sieve (MPTT-24) at identifying patients needing life-saving interventions, it is to be removed from UK practice in 2022. Whilst the optimum method of secondary triage is still to be decided, in the interim, UK practice is to repeat the MITT assessment (using the modified triage sieve based on the MPTT-24) and to combine this with a senior clinician review.

15.11 Summary

- Triage is the first step in the hierarchy of medical support at a major incident
- It is a dynamic process, starting with the sieve at the site where patients are found, moving via a physiological and anatomical triage sorting process in the CCS (triage sort) and continuing on arrival at the receiving hospital through to the point of definitive care
- Folding labels are the best labels available for dynamic triage

15.12 Reference

Vassallo J, Smith JE, Wallis LA. Major incident triage and the implementation of a new triage tool, the MPTT-24. *J R Army Med Corps* 2018; 164: 103–106.

CHAPTER 16
Treatment

Learning outcomes

After reading this chapter you will be able to:
- Describe who should carry out treatment at the scene
- Detail where treatment is carried out at the scene
- Describe what treatments are carried out at the scene
- Discuss how much treatment is carried out at the scene

16.1 Introduction

The treatment phase is the second step in medical support at the scene. The aim is the minimal necessary intervention that results in live casualties who can be transported to hospital (or other suitable healthcare facility) for definitive treatment in a timely and humane way. During a major incident, a large number of people will become involved in the treatment of the injured and ill; ranging from other casualties and concerned bystanders, who may have medical training, to specialist clinicians. A key aspect of triage is the identification of patients who require immediate treatment at the scene and as a result, triage should precede treatment when numbers of patients exceed numbers of clinicians able to treat them.

Key point

The aim of treatment is to undertake the minimal necessary intervention to ensure the patients are stable enough to be transported from the scene to the treatment facility.

16.2 Who carries out treatment at the scene?

The public/bystanders

Very basic forms of treatment may be started in the initial stages of the incident by survivors involved in the incident (who may be injured themselves) and by bystanders who were close to the incident when it occurred. Some of those providing this immediate treatment may be trained in basic first aid and some may be healthcare professionals. These actions may be life saving. However, this immediate intervention will be uncoordinated, lacking the appropriate kit and equipment, and will not be able to deal effectively with a large number of casualties.

Key point

Initial first aid may be provided by other survivors and bystanders.

Major Incident Medical Management and Support: The Practical Approach at the Scene, Fourth Edition.
Edited by Tony Gleeson and Kevin Mackway-Jones.
© 2023 John Wiley & Sons Ltd. Published 2023 by John Wiley & Sons Ltd.

First aiders

It is only when the emergency services begin to arrive that large numbers of people trained in first aid are likely to be found at the scene. All police and fire service personnel receive instruction in life-saving first aid; furthermore, some non-health emergency services carry advanced life support equipment and increasingly carry blast/haemorrhage control equipment (for example, combat application tourniquets and blast dressings). Once their initial responsibilities have been discharged, and as part of a joint, coordinated tasking, all emergency services personnel may become involved in basic treatment.

> **Key point**
>
> Once their initial tasks have been accomplished, other emergency services can assist in first aid.

Ambulance service

In the UK, the ambulance service has overall responsibility for providing treatment at all incidents outside the hospital. The skills within this service range from first aid to advanced life support. Allocation of tasks should reflect skill level.

Specialist medical response

Medical staff at the scene will come from different backgrounds, and may include doctors, nurses and specialist-role (in the UK, 'critical care') paramedics. Their primary role is to complement the ambulance service and provide more advanced treatments. These providers are often trained to work as self-contained teams (for example Helicopter Emergency Medical Services (HEMS) and Medical Emergency Response Incident Teams (MERIT)). In local planning for major incidents, consideration should be given to employ these personnel at the incident site in their pre-established teams and to direct them to tasks that best fit their normal operations.

Potential roles include:

1. Managing a single severely injured/unwell patient in the Casualty Clearing Station (CCS).
2. Transport of a single patient to hospital (potentially out-of-region to a specialist centre if HEMS).
3. Medical management of a trapped patient (analgesia/sedation/anaesthesia and, rarely, amputation).
4. Undertaking mass triage in a defined area of responsibility.

Other specialist providers may attend the incident as individuals, for example in the UK as a British Association for Immediate Care Schemes (BASICS) responder. Local agreement should be in place as to how best utilise these personnel after they have initially reported to the Medical Incident Officer (MIO), but may include medical incident command roles (where appropriately trained) and providing care in the CCS. In the UK, all specialist providers attending a major incident should be suitably qualified and experienced in pre-hospital care and have the correct personal protective equipment (PPE). In other systems, the role utilisation of specialist providers will depend on their training and experience of working safely pre-hospital – it may be that they are restricted to the relatively hazard-free CCS.

16.3 Hierarchy of medical support

It is absolutely essential that those managing the health service response remember the hierarchy of medical support (Box 16.1).

Box 16.1 Hierarchy of medical support

- **T**riage
- **T**reatment
- **T**ransport

Triage

In order to achieve the best overall outcome for the casualties, triage must precede both treatment and transport. Once triage has been carried out, then the limited advanced treatment capability can be directed to those casualties who have the greatest need. Rescuers with a lower skill level can be used to look after casualties with less immediate problems.

Treatment

Where is treatment carried out?

In the initial stages, before the medical response becomes structured, the vast majority of first aid measures will be provided at the site of the incident by bystanders. These first aid measures will be carried out within the first few minutes after the incident has occurred.

Once the emergency services arrive, a command and control structure will be put in place (Figure 16.1) and the focus will be on treatment in a Casualty Clearing Station (CCS). This is a more suitable environment for advanced procedures to take place and allows clearer command and control oversight.

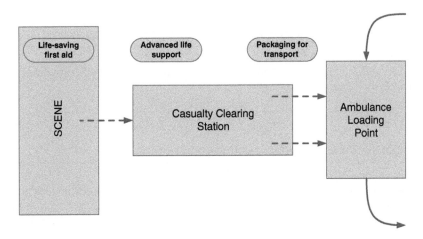

Figure 16.1 Treatment at the scene

There may be some merit in moving those with minor injuries to a 'place of safety' in the first instance, where they can receive any necessary first aid before undergoing secondary triage and disposal to either the Survivor Reception Centre or acute hospital/other appropriate healthcare facility. However, unless this 'place of safety' is located immediately adjacent to the CCS this method reduces the ability of ambulance commanders to maintain control, and increases risk to casualties who may develop a requirement to undergo life-saving intervention. It is therefore better to process all casualties through the CCS, and where appropriate move them to a Survivor Reception Centre after further triage. Consideration should also be given to the use of other, non-acute hospital/healthcare facilities (primary care centres, walk-in-centres, minor injury units, etc.) for casualties with minor injuries in order to reduce the burden on hospitals.

In certain circumstances, treatment will take place at the site. Casualties who are trapped may need advanced measures (typically analgesia, sedation and, rarely, amputation); these will need to be provided *in situ*.

How much treatment is carried out?

The aim of treatment at the scene of an incident is to ensure that casualties are well enough to undertake the journey to a facility where they can be fully assessed and treated, and no more. This is in keeping with the overall treatment aim of minimal necessary intervention.

The amount of treatment needed before transport often reflects the triage category. A walking patient who has been categorised *T3, delayed* may be moved to a healthcare facility without receiving any treatment at all. On the other hand, a casualty with a compromised airway who has been categorised *T1, immediate* may require considerable input at the scene in order to make transportation as safe as possible.

What treatment is carried out?

Virtually any treatment can be provided pre-hospital. However, this does not mean that all treatments should be provided at the scene (whether at a major incident or not). The aim of treatment remains the safe transportation of the casualty to hospital in a timely and humane way; therefore, the amount of treatment should be limited to that which ensures that this is possible – it is always preferable to treat patients in a hospital than casualties at the scene.

> **Key point**
>
> Where possible, it is always preferable to treat patients in a hospital than casualties pre-hospital.

Overall, medical management will be optimal if treatment is kept at this level. If too little is done, casualties will die unnecessarily on the way to hospital. If too much is done, then time and resources that could have been spent on other casualties will have been wasted. Treatments at the scene are therefore likely to be limited to those concerned with problems of the airway, breathing and circulation. Other treatment measures may be necessary – up to and including amputation for extrication, although this will be very rare.

> **Key point**
>
> Most treatment at a major incident will be directed towards airway, breathing and circulation.

The treatment that health service staff provide should remain within the limits of their competence. Health personnel will work much better doing a job similar to their day-to-day practice.

> **Key point**
>
> Health service personnel at the scene should not operate outside their skill level.

Treatments at the scene generally fall into two categories: immediate life-saving intervention (LSI) and the treatment of pain (by analgesia and dressings/splints). What constitutes an LSI during the definitive (hospital) care of a patient during a major incident has recently been defined via expert consensus (Vassallo et al., 2016). Arguably, only 20 of the 32 LSIs identified are appropriate, or likely to be available, pre-hospital at a major incident, as shown in Table 16.1.

Table 16.1 Consensus-derived life-saving interventions during a major incident, suitable for the pre-hospital phase

Number	Category	Intervention
1	Airway	Intubation for impending airway obstruction
2		Intubation for actual airway obstruction
3		Surgical airway for impending airway obstruction
4		Surgical airway for actual airway obstruction
5	Breathing	Needle thoracocentesis
6		Finger thoracostomy
7		Tube thoracostomy (chest drain)
8		Application of a chest seal
9		Positive pressure ventilation
10	Circulation	Application of a tourniquet for haemorrhage control
11		Use of a haemostatic agent for haemorrhage control
12		Insertion of an intraosseous needle for resuscitation
13		Administration of tranexamic acid
14		Application of a pelvic binder
15		ALS/ACLS for a peri-arrest patient
16		ALS/ACLS for an arrest patient
17	Other	Spinal injury precautions (immobilisation/careful handling)
18		Administration of seizure-terminating medication
19		Correction of low blood glucose
20		Administration of chemical antidotes

Within 'airway', there are other more basic interventions that may also be considered as LSIs in this setting, for example, manual opening of the airway, and the insertion of oropharyngeal, nasopharyngeal or supraglottic (for example laryngeal mask airway (LMA)/iGel) airways.

The use of blood and blood products (for example, thawed fresh frozen plasma and spray-dried plasma) is increasing in pre-hospital care. As of 2019, the Israeli Defence Force use fresh whole blood as their primary resuscitation fluid in traumatic haemorrhage, the US military have started a program of far-forward low-titre O whole blood (LTOWB), Norwegian HEMS units carry either whole blood or units of packed red blood cells and fresh frozen plasma, and a number of UK HEMS carry units of packed red blood cells and or spray-dried plasma. It is therefore possible that blood and blood products will be available at the scene of major incidents. However, this is an evolving area of pre-hospital care, and these resuscitation fluids are unlikely to be available in large quantities in the near future. The future direction of this capability is likely to be focused around pre-screened emergency donor panels for the rapid collection of LTOWB, such as the current 'Purple Alert' system in San Antonio, Texas, USA, that can be activated during a major incident or other times of increased demand.

Transport

An important component in treatment is the packaging of the patient for safe transport to hospital. Measures to prevent exacerbation of spinal injuries are an integral part of packaging for transport. For this reason, the Loading Point is situated directly outside, or as near as possible to, the Casualty Clearing Station.

It is essential that the ambulance, paramedical, nursing and medical personnel who are sent to the scene of a major incident are appropriately competent. It is totally unacceptable for health staff attending a major incident response to be either untrained or poorly skilled. Table 16.2 summarises the areas in which responding staff should have competence.

Table 16.2 Areas of essential competence for responders

Responder	Competence required
Ambulance officer	Incident management
Ambulance paramedic	Primary triage, trauma care, life support
Doctor	Primary and secondary triage, advanced trauma care, advanced life support, minor injury assessment
Nurse	Primary triage, advanced trauma nursing care, life support, minor injury assessment
Critical care paramedic	Primary triage, advanced trauma care, life support, minor injury assessment

Local highlights: Expected qualifications of responders

16.4 Clinical responsibility

The issue of where clinical responsibility rests is difficult to resolve. It is clearly the responsibility of the Ambulance Incident Commander to ensure that there are enough ambulance personnel at the scene supported by enough equipment to perform their role to best practice standards. Equally, the Medical Commander has a responsibility to identify the right number and skill mix of clinical personnel needed to support the ambulance service. If this has been achieved, then individual clinicians must take responsibility for their own actions.

16.5 Summary

- The first treatment delivered is likely to be basic first aid from unskilled people
- Emergency service personnel are all trained in life-saving first aid
- The ambulance service has responsibility for treatment at the scene
- Attention to airway, breathing and circulation is most often all that is required at the scene
- All health staff attending major incidents should have current competency at the appropriate skill level

CHAPTER 17
Transport

Learning outcomes

After reading this chapter you will be able to:
- Describe how the Casualty Clearing Station and other areas set up to facilitate evacuation and transportation
- Discuss what decisions about transportation need to be made
- List the methods of transportation that are available

17.1 Introduction

Transport is the third step in medical support at a major incident (Box 17.1). Both triage and treatment decisions will have an effect on transportation. To a large degree, the order of evacuation, the destination and the mode of transportation will be dictated by early command decisions made jointly between the Ambulance Commander and Medical Advisor/ Commander. The senior clinician of the treating team and the Casualty Clearing Station Officer will also be involved in the decision-making process.

Box 17.1 The hierarchy of medical support

- **T**riage
- **T**reatment
- **T**ransport

As discussed in Chapter 2, one of the primary tasks of the health service command and control structure is to ensure that the movement of patients is as efficient as possible. To achieve this, close attention needs to be paid to the organisation of transportation both at the scene and beyond. The structure of the treatment and evacuation areas is crucial, as are decisions regarding evacuation methods. Furthermore, the officers responsible for transportation need to have the ability to be flexible about methods of transport and the order of evacuation, if the best use is to be made of resources available.

17.2 Organisation

Casualties requiring evacuation from the scene will not necessarily arrive at the Casualty Clearing Station (CCS) in priority order. This may change the form of transport required at various times throughout the incident.

Chain of transport

Once a major incident has been declared, ambulance resources will be deployed to the scene from a variety of locations. It is imperative that a preferred access route is established early, which is both safe and also delivers resources to a single point. This will expedite the arrival of resources for the initial Ambulance Incident Commander. Once emergency service Operational

Major Incident Medical Management and Support: The Practical Approach at the Scene, Fourth Edition.
Edited by Tony Gleeson and Kevin Mackway-Jones.
© 2023 John Wiley & Sons Ltd. Published 2023 by John Wiley & Sons Ltd.

Commanders are on scene and the Forward Control Point or Forward Command is established, access and egress routes through the outer cordon will be agreed. The 'ambulance circuit' will then be used by all ambulance resources as they arrive at the agreed parking point and leave the loading point en route to receiving hospitals.

Once in position, the Ambulance Parking Point Officer will hold vehicles at the Parking Point and will dispatch them as required. A range of vehicles may be available and they will be matched to patient needs.

Once called forward, vehicles will proceed to the Ambulance Loading Point (which should be as close to the CCS as possible) and will load their assigned casualties. The Ambulance Loading Officer will inform the crew of the patient's condition, ongoing treatment requirements en route and destination. This will be recorded by the Ambulance Loading Officer. Once released from the Loading Point, ambulances will proceed around the circuit to an exit point at the outer cordon, then to their destination. This system ensures that both the number and nature of vehicles at the Loading Point is optimised.

A schematic representation of the ambulance circuit is shown in Figure 17.1.

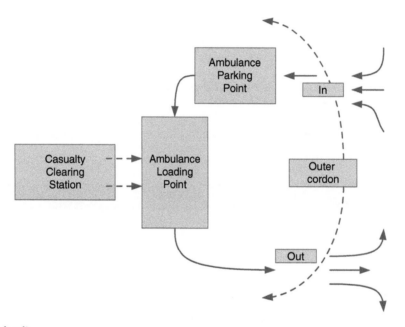

Figure 17.1 Ambulance circuit

Casualty flow

Priority 3 casualties have initially been triaged as such because they are walking. This group of casualties do not, as a matter of course, go to the CCS but are directed in the short term to a place of safety prior to the establishment of a Survivor Reception Centre. The Ambulance Incident Commander must, however, ensure that an appropriate medical resource is assigned to this location to carry out secondary triage (triage sort). This is to reassess the patients and to ensure that there is an available clinical resource if any priority 3 patient's condition deteriorates. The schemes detailed in Figures 17.2 and 17.3 show possible casualty flows from incident site through to receiving hospital.

In the first scheme (Figure 17.2), patients who are priority 1 (immediate) and priority 2 (urgent) are moved to the Casualty Clearing Station and from there to the Loading Point.

If the expectant category is in use, then regular re-triage must take place to confirm their priority status. Priority 4 patients should be evacuated after all priority 1 patients have been dealt with (Figure 17.3). The level of care required for this group may be beyond that available at certain points in the incident. In the second evacuation scheme, the priority 3 (delayed) patients bypass the CCS and are transported to a receiving hospital/facility. Ideally however, these patients should have secondary triage (triage sort) before leaving the scene, as this will better identify patients at risk of deterioration en route and allow for stabilisation prior to transport. Those at risk of deterioration would be sent to the CCS for stabilisation prior to transport.

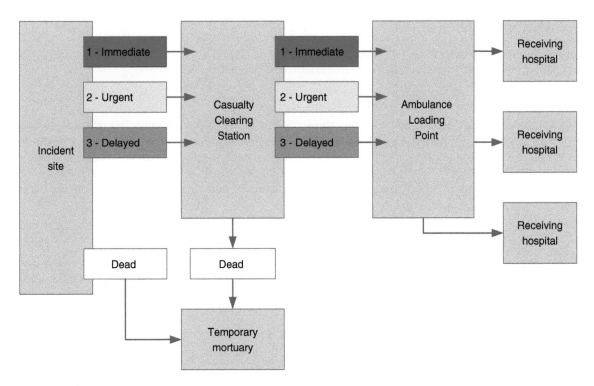

Figure 17.2 Evacuation scheme 1

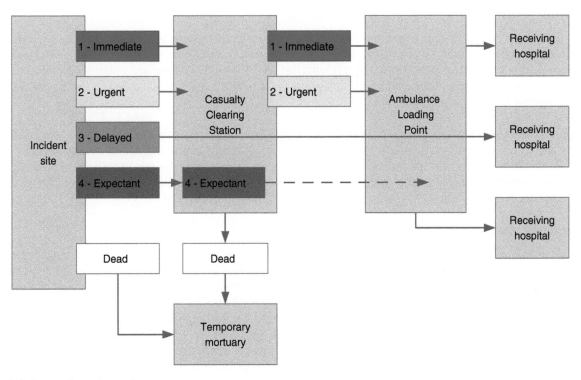

Figure 17.3 Evacuation scheme 2

17.3 Evacuation decisions

There are three key decisions to be made before a particular patient is moved from the scene. The first concerns priority for evacuation, the second treatment and packaging for evacuation, and the third is destination.

Priority for evacuation

Generally, the priority for evacuation will be exactly the same as priority after treatment. The triage sieve and triage sort techniques described in Chapter 15 can be used to determine priorities in the CCS. There may be multiple casualties within the same triage category after sieve and sort have been used and other forms of triage may have to be used to determine priority for evacuation. Casualty Clearing Officers may have to use additional criteria such as the availability of suitable transport and the capacity of vehicles leaving for particular destinations to decide the order of evacuation.

> **Key point**
>
> Although triage category in the evacuation area is reached using standard triage principles, other criteria will have to be taken into account when deciding the exact order that patients leave the scene.

Treatment and packaging

The correct amount of treatment is that necessary to ensure safe transportation of a casualty to hospital, or, if stabilisation is not possible, the amount which will give the casualty the best chance of surviving to reach hospital.

> **Key point**
>
> Treatment and packaging should be limited to that necessary to allow safe transport.

Destination

It is the responsibility of the ambulance service with advice from the Medical Commander/Advisor to decide which hospitals are to be used as receiving hospitals. Local major incident plans may specify which hospitals should receive which categories of patients, in particular when hospitals form a Major Trauma Network. The Medical Commander/Advisor at the Tactical level must establish how many patients of each triage category can be accepted by each hospital. This should be reviewed on a regular basis as the incident continues.

In larger urban areas, where there is a choice of destinations, it is better to select patients for direct transfer to specialist facilities at the scene of the incident. Patients with multiple severe injuries should be transferred directly to major trauma centres, providing there are suitable transport resources available to facilitate the transfer, especially if distances are long. The Medical Commander/Advisor may also contribute to decisions about which patients are suitable for direct transfer to other specialist units, for example patients with severe burns may be sent to regional burns units.

Predetermined plans to receive casualties

In larger urban centres with trauma networks in place and a choice of hospitals to receive, there is an increasing move towards having a predetermined allocation of numbers of patients to go to hospital facilities on the declaration of a major incident. A large urban trauma centre may agree to receive a certain number of priority 1s in the first 2 hours of an incident, a trauma unit would accept a certain number of priority 2s in a similar 2-hour period and other emergency departments priority 3s during the same time frame. The advantage of this is that the Medical Commander knows that a particular receiving hospital has the plans in place to receive these patients without having to worry about overloading the receiving sites. Clearly this needs to be planned and exercised before any incident takes place. This system was in place and utilised during the Manchester Arena Bombing in May 2017 and post incident there were only two interhospital transfers.

Key point

Casualties requiring specialist centres should be transported to them directly from the scene:
RIGHT PATIENT, RIGHT PLACE, RIGHT TIME – FIRST TIME.

17.4 Methods of transportation

Emergency ambulances

The usual method of transportation in everyday practice is an emergency ambulance. Such vehicles are specifically designed to enable safe transport of the seriously ill and injured, and have many facilities for the provision of advanced life support en route. In a major incident, when normal health service responses are overwhelmed, there may not be enough of these vehicles, and other methods of transportation need to be considered.

Other land vehicles

Three key elements must be considered by the Ambulance Incident Commander when transportation needs and possibilities are being assessed (Box 17.2). Firstly, what **capacity** is needed and what capacity does each potential vehicle have? Secondly, what is the **availability** of each of the potential vehicles? Thirdly, the **suitability** of the various potential vehicles for the task in hand? This latter decision needs to be based on an assessment of the speed, safety, reliability and levels of equipment. A standard emergency ambulance, for example, will be unsuitable for rough terrain when access roads are limited (unless it is four-wheel drive), and specialist all-terrain vehicles may have to be used to rescue casualties to the CCS but are unlikely to be able to convey to hospital. A helicopter may need to be considered if the incident scene is very remote.

Box 17.2 Criteria for selecting transportation for patients

- **C**apacity
- **A**vailability
- **S**uitability

The transport of priority 3 patients may be undertaken by non-ambulance vehicles, the use of police personnel carriers or commandeering public transport such as buses may be considered. More seriously ill or injured patients who need to be transported on stretchers are more difficult to transport in non-specialist vehicles. Patient transport ambulances fitted for stretchers may be suitable for priority 2 (urgent) patients. Escorts with suitable equipment and medical training must accompany casualties being transported on non-medical platforms (for example buses) in case of deterioration en route to the hospital.

Helicopters

The use of helicopters in a major incident is likely to bring multiple benefits however needs to be considered against the potential hazards. Dedicated Helicopter Emergency Medical Service (HEMS) aircraft can usually only carry a single stretcher patient and the provision of helicopters for mass transport is limited. Other aircraft, such as those that can be provided by the armed forces, are rarely fitted for stretcher carrying, and vary in both capacity and suitability. Helicopters are most suitable for the deployment of specialist medical teams and when rapid transfer to a specialist centre is required, the road infrastructure is disrupted or the terrain is unsuitable for ambulances.

In other circumstances, the disadvantages may outweigh the advantages. Multiple aircraft landing at the incident site will require coordination and a suitable helicopter landing site will have to be identified. In some areas the lack of a primary helicopter landing site at the hospital may mean that a secondary ambulance transfer from a distant landing site (such as a school playing field) will be necessary, this will be challenging if ambulance resources are already depleted responding to the incident

> **Key point**
>
> Helicopters are most suitable for deploying specialist medical teams or when rapid transfer over a distance to a specialist centre is required.

Other possibilities

In particular circumstances the use of other types of transport, such as boat or train, may be considered. For instance, many major airports are extremely well connected to the rail network. If the area is isolated from the main receiving hospitals or if local hospitals are likely to be unable to cope with the numbers of casualties, then it may be advantageous to move some casualties en masse by rail and re-triage them on arrival at a station close to other hospitals.

Self-presentation

Historically it has been observed that in a number of major incidents, varying numbers of casualties have self-presented themselves to hospitals, bypassing the traditional emergency medical services. Hospitals must therefore be aware of this and expect to receive patients who will, by definition, not have been triaged and, in the case of CBRN events, will not have decontaminated prior to their arrival at hospital.

17.5 Summary

- Transportation is the third step in medical support at major incidents
- Effective organisation of both the ambulance circuit and the flow of patients is vital if evacuation is to proceed smoothly
- The order of patient evacuation depends on both triage category and other factors
- Emergency ambulances form the mainstay of transport capacity
- Other vehicles may need to be used when the circumstances are appropriate
- Helicopters may play a part and can be invaluable in particular circumstances

CHAPTER 18
Responsibility for the dead

Learning outcomes

After reading this chapter you will be able to:
- Describe the process of pronouncing death
- Discuss the importance of labelling the dead
- Discuss the processes around moving the dead
- Describe the issues to consider in establishing a temporary mortuary
- Describe the processes used to identify the dead

18.1 Introduction

Major incidents invariably will result in casualties who die. Some will die at the incident site, some in the Casualty Clearing Station (CCS) and others at hospital. There may even be some who die en route to the CCS or hospital (despite the best efforts of clinicians to stabilise for transport). The health service has an obligation to preserve evidence as much as possible, to facilitate the enquiry that will occur after the incident and, as such, it is important to be clear and to have a plan to deal with each of these scenarios. Dead casualties should not be moved at the scene of the incident unless they are obstructing access to the living or if there is a risk of destruction of the body (for example in a fire). If movement is required, photographs of the positions of the dead prior to movement should be taken. Formal identification of the dead by the police service may be reliant on personal effects and the health service should ensure that all personnel effects belonging to the individual are carefully sealed and labelled in bags and kept with the individual.

18.2 Pronouncing death

At the scene of a major incident it would be usual to regard a casualty as dead if the casualty does not breathe for 10 seconds when their airway is opened during primary triage (the triage sieve), or the injuries are of such severity that they are incompatible with life. Any health professional who has been taught the triage sieve algorithm can therefore 'diagnose' death. The process of formally 'pronouncing life extinct' has typically been the role of a medical practitioner at a later stage in the incident. In the company of a police officer, a medical practitioner will need to carry out a more thorough conventional examination to formally pronounce that death has occurred. This would include confirming the presence of apnoea, asystole (no palpable pulse) and fixed dilated pupils. Since the death is sudden and typically unexpected, the case will be subject to a Coroner's investigation being carried out, providing a 'death certificate' and defining the cause of death. This will usually involve a post-mortem examination and require an inquest.

Major Incident Medical Management and Support: The Practical Approach at the Scene, Fourth Edition.
Edited by Tony Gleeson and Kevin Mackway-Jones.
© 2023 John Wiley & Sons Ltd. Published 2023 by John Wiley & Sons Ltd.

18.3 Labelling the dead

It is important to clearly label the dead using a triage card system. Failure to do this may result in rescue personnel repeatedly revisiting and reassessing a body, wasting valuable clinical time when resuscitation capacity is limited. On diagnosis of death, a 'Dead' triage label should be fastened to the patient in a clearly visible position. The Medical Incident Adviser may appoint a medical practitioner to work with the police to formally pronounce death, label the bodies at scene and, in collaboration with the police service, establish a Body Holding Area. When this is completed, the label should include the date, time, name of the medical practitioner and the signature and police number of the police officer witnessing the process.

18.4 Moving the dead

A major incident will often be regarded by the police as a potential scene of crime. The dead form part of the forensic evidence. The position they are found in may be important, both to the criminal investigation and also to determine identity. For these reasons, the dead (or body parts) should not be moved without both police authorisation and appropriate documentation. Each separate body part should be labelled without assumption as to which body a part belongs to. If it is necessary to move a body to gain access to the living, then the urgency of the situation should be assessed. **Saving life has precedence over the preservation of forensic evidence**, therefore the movement of a body without permission for the delivery of life-saving treatment to a live casualty is justifiable.

Reasons for moving the dead:

- To gain access to the living and aid in their rescue
- To prevent destruction of a body or body part by fire or chemical

The police should be notified as soon as possible. The original position should be recorded as clearly as possible and a record should be made of where the body (or part) has been moved to. In some exceptional circumstances, it may be necessary to dismember a body, perhaps to gain essential rapid access to a live casualty. A description of injuries to the body (possibly photographic) will be important, together with a clear outline of the actions undertaken by the rescuers.

18.5 Temporary mortuary

When a body or body part is moved from the scene (possibly via a Body Holding Area), it is transported to a predetermined specialist hospital mortuary where a forensic pathologist can examine it. In smaller incidents, where the number of fatalities is limited, the Coroner may decide that a local hospital mortuary with the capacity would be appropriate for this. However, in larger incidents, particularly when there is the additional problem of fragmentation of bodies, a different and larger venue will be chosen and a temporary mortuary may be established. The decision as to whether a temporary mortuary is established is usually made because of the need to identify bodies when identification is difficult (fragmentation, burns etc.). The police will have total control of the temporary mortuary.

The medical issues to consider when choosing a temporary mortuary are:

- Capacity
- Low ambient temperature
- Privacy and security
- Adequate sanitation and waste handling
- Changing and rest areas for staff
- Facility for x-ray and other forensic pathology investigations
- Link to the Family Assistance Centre and Welfare Centre

For most incidents, potential temporary mortuaries have often been identified at the planning stage. Large public buildings such as sports halls or aircraft hangers are often appropriate. A temporary facility may be constructed specifically for the purpose and be removed when this work is completed. If an incident occurs some distance from a designated area, a Body Holding Area may be set up at the scene. This must be out of sight of the media and the public and should preferably be protected from the elements. Refrigerated lorries might be an option to consider. All live casualties should be evacuated from the scene before transport is used for the dead.

Examples of incidents that have warranted the establishment of temporary mortuaries

6 March 1987 – Zeebrugge Ferry disaster
21 December 1988 – Lockerbie bombing
7 July 2005 – London bombing
22 May 2017 – Manchester Arena bombing

18.6 Identifying the dead

This is the responsibility of the police. It may be possible to identify the individual from clothing, personal documentation or personal effects. Caution must be taken as a coat or other garment may have been placed over a body to provide some dignity and may not belong to that body. Personal effects such as rings, watches or wallets must not be removed from bodies for safekeeping since these may also be clues to the identity of the deceased. Because of the possible uncertainty, the identification of a body by simple means such as personal effects is rarely sufficient and techniques such as forensic dentistry and DNA matching may also be used. Information on the identity of people who may have been involved in an incident is often available to friends and relatives. Typically, a Casualty Bureau will be established by the police (neighbouring police force area) to collate information relating to a body (clothes, jewellery, distinguishing marks, etc.). Specific proformas and questioning systems are used to query contacts to help determine the identity of the dead. However, in some cases and as previously mentioned, the only method of identification will be through dental records or DNA.

18.7 Summary

- Dealing correctly with those casualties who die at the scene of a major incident is important to facilitate identification by the police
- The health service has an obligation under the common goals of all responding services to facilitate an enquiry post-incident by preserving evidence. It is important that the clinician has a clear understanding of how the dead are managed at the scene to achieve this goal
- Preservation of evidence is important but should not compromise the care of the living

PART VI
Special incidents

CHAPTER 19
Hazardous materials and CBRNe incidents

Learning outcomes

After reading this chapter you will be able to:
- Discuss the actions required at hazardous materials incidents by responding agencies
- Describe the command structure at an incident involving hazardous materials
- Define the zones and cordons at hazardous material incidents

---

19.1 Introduction

Plans that deal with the consequences of incidents involving hazardous materials (HazMat) and chemical, biological, radiological, nuclear and explosive (CBRNe) materials have been developed using knowledge gained from live incidents and multiagency exercises. In general, plans are suitable for both HazMat and CBRNe events.

1. **HazMat incident:** An *accidental* release of a substance, agent or material that results in illness or injury, the denial of access to an area or the interruption of the food chain.
2. **CBRNe incidents:** These are usually *deliberate*. The term covers a distinct range of hazards:
   - *Chemical*: Poisoning or injury caused by chemical substances, including chemical warfare agents, or misuse of legitimate but harmful household or industrial chemicals
   - *Biological*: Illnesses caused by the deliberate release of dangerous bacteria, viruses, fungi or toxins (for example the plant toxin, ricin)
   - *Radiological*: Illnesses caused by exposure to harmful radioactive materials, possibly inhaled or ingested in food or drink
   - *Nuclear*: The explosion of a nuclear device causes widespread effects due to blast, heat and large amounts of harmful radiation
   - *Explosives*: The use of explosive devices to disperse CBRNe agents

Irrespective of the particular responsibilities of organisations and agencies responding to the incident, coordinated effective multiagency activity is necessary to achieve the following:

- Preserve and protect lives
- Mitigate and minimise the impact of an incident
- Inform the public and maintain public confidence
- Prevent, deter and detect crime
- Assist an early return to normality

Other important common objectives involve managing the health and safety of all those responding to the incident, safeguarding the environment, facilitating judicial, public, technical, or other inquiries and, finally, evaluating the response and identifying lessons to be learned.

Major Incident Medical Management and Support: The Practical Approach at the Scene, Fourth Edition.
Edited by Tony Gleeson and Kevin Mackway-Jones.
© 2023 John Wiley & Sons Ltd. Published 2023 by John Wiley & Sons Ltd.

19.2 Roles and responsibilities of responding agencies

Ambulance service

The ambulance service has the principal responsibility for pre-hospital triage and decontamination of contaminated casualties at Hazmat/CBRNe incidents. However, all responding agencies will collaborate to ensure that the risk to casualties from continuing exposure to the hazard is properly controlled. The ambulance service will have specially trained responders with the appropriate personal protective equipment (PPE) and equipment to carry out these tasks. In the UK these are called the Hazardous Area Response Team (HART).

Fire and rescue service

The core functions of the fire and rescue service (FRS) are saving life, protecting property and the environment from fire and other emergencies, and providing humanitarian services. The management of operations within the inner cordon is normally delegated to the FRS, including the safety of all personnel working within it. Recovery or rescue from within the inner cordon will, in all but exceptional circumstances, be the responsibility of the FRS, however specialist resources from other agencies may support this.

If circumstances require the implementation of mass decontamination or other form of decontamination, then the ambulance service may request that the FRS assist in the implementation of these procedures.

Police service

The police service undertake the overall coordination of activity at the scene of a major incident, which will include all incidents that require the decontamination of people exposed to CBRNe material. The police often have specialist officers trained in the use of CBRNe PPE. These officers will deploy where required within the contaminated area if operationally viable and safe to do so.

19.3 Cordons and zones

Initial cordon

The initial cordon is temporarily established by the first wave of unprotected emergency responders – before any detailed scene assessment or any other scientific analysis has been conducted. It provides an initial means of containing the problem and adds an element of control to the incident.

Inner cordon

The inner cordon encompasses both the hot and warm zones. It must provide a secure environment for the emergency services and other agencies to work within.

Inner cordon gateway

A controlled route into the hot zone where entry control processes and safe undressing procedures can be managed.

Outer cordon

The outer cordon designates the controlled area into which unauthorised access is not permitted. It encompasses the hot, warm and cold zones (Figure 19.1).

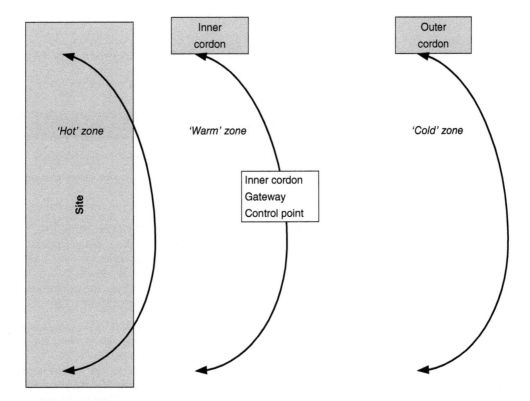

Figure 19.1 Contamination zones

Cold zone

This is the uncontaminated area between the inner cordon and the outer cordon.

Warm zone

This is the area uncontaminated by the initial release of a substance, which becomes contaminated by the movement of people or vehicles.

Hot zone

This is the contaminated area (or areas) where the initial release occurred or disperses to. It will be the area likely to pose an immediate threat to the health and safety of all those located within it and is the area of greatest risk.

19.4 Safety

Recognition of potential safety issues is important and a high index of suspicion should be maintained. The STEP 1-2-3 Plus tool shown in Box 19.1 is designed to facilitate early recognition and therefore to maximise safety.

Box 19.1 STEP 1-2-3 Plus

Step 1	*One* casualty, incapacitated with no obvious reason	• Approach using normal procedures
Step 2	*Two* casualties, incapacitated with no obvious reason	• Approach with caution using normal procedures • Consider all options • Report on arrival and update Control
Step 3	*Three or more* casualties, in close proximity, incapacitated with no obvious reason	• DO NOT APPROACH THE SCENE • Withdraw from the scene to a place of safety • Contain the scene • Provide a situation report • Isolate yourself if you are contaminated • SEND FOR SPECIALIST HELP

Plus		• Follow the local CBRNe response algorithm:
		  • **REMOVE** those affected from the contaminated area (get people away from the scene, ideally uphill/upwind)
		  • **REMOVE** outer layer of clothing (ask casualties to remove outer clothing as this can remove up to 80% of the contaminant)
		  • **REMOVE** contaminant from the skin using dry absorbent material to brush off or soak up (ask casualties to use dry decontamination as the default process – rinse off with water if the skin is itching or burning)
		• Communicate and advise – give immediate medical advice and reassurance that help is on the way

---

There may also be other signs, which might be useful in confirming a release and going some way to identifying the substance involved. If a problem has already been identified using STEP 1-2-3 Plus then no additional signs should be sought. Equally, if other signs are noted before STEP 1-2-3 Plus, withdrawal should be immediate and Control must be informed.

Other signs are:

- Dead animals/birds/fish in large numbers
- Lack of insect life: dead insects in surrounding area
- Physical symptoms: numerous individuals experiencing water-like blisters, pinpoint pupils, choking, respiratory distress or rashes
- Mass casualties: numerous individuals presenting with health problems ranging from nausea and disorientation to respiratory distress, usually with sudden onset
- Unusual liquid droplets: surfaces may have oily droplets, water surfaces may have an oily film
- Unusual appearance: trees, lawns, shrubs and bushes may be discoloured, withered or dead
- Unexplained odours: ranging from fruity or flowery to sharp/pungent to garlic/horseradish to new-mown hay. It is important that the odour is out of character with the surroundings
- Low-lying clouds or fog-like conditions that are not explained by prevailing weather conditions

As well as injury and illnesses in people, all of the above features pose the threat of environmental contamination.

19.5 Treatment

When people are exposed to hazardous substances, these can become lodged on their clothing, skin and hair and present a continuing health risk for themselves and their immediate contacts. It is important, therefore, that safe and effective early decontamination (removal of the contaminant to prevent further exposure of the contaminated individual and to minimise the spread of the contaminant) be undertaken. However, decontamination is not an inevitable response to HazMat or CBRNe events. Whether or not to initiate decontamination procedures will depend on the initial assessment of the nature of the event by first responders and subsequently by trained ambulance service specialists.

Decisions on whether to decontaminate and which decontamination option(s) to pursue will depend greatly on the circumstances of the incident and on the findings of the operational hazard and risk assessments carried out by the emergency services at the scene. Responsibility for these decisions will rest with the Ambulance Commander in consultation with the Fire and Police Commander. This includes consideration of the different needs and options for decontamination of those affected, who are either injured or uninjured, and for those who exhibit or develop signs and symptoms of exposure or contamination, as opposed to those who do not.

Decontamination procedures (for people, equipment, property or the environment) are not new and are routinely carried out by emergency service responders dealing with incidents involving hazardous substances. In most instances, this involves the responders themselves having their protective clothing decontaminated using cold or warm water applied manually or through simple showering devices.

For many incidents, the earliest contacts with contaminated casualties will be emergency services personnel involved in their rescue, triage and treatment. In addition to direct physical contact with the contaminant, these responders might also risk exposure to airborne substances that are re-aerosolised or vaporised (commonly referred to as 'off-gassing') from the contaminated person.

Decontamination of casualties should be managed as part of a multiagency response. This applies to all situations, minor or major, where the contamination poses a threat to the health of contaminated casualties or their contacts. Further action might be required by other responding organisations for the decontamination of exposed facilities and environments and of any surfaces with which a contaminated casualty has come into contact.

Hierarchy of categories

Decontamination can take several forms ranging from improvised decontamination by people responding to an immediate and necessary need, through to full and comprehensive decontamination. However, the initial response is very important and can be carried out by non-specialist responders.

Initial response

Having identified the likelihood of casualties being contaminated with a CBRNe agent using STEP 1-2-3, it is important to utilise the 'Plus' part of the process by initiating a Remove, Remove, Remove response.

Using caution, and keeping a safe distance to avoid exposure, contaminated casualties should be advised to:

- **Remove** themselves from the immediate area to avoid further contamination
- **Remove** outer clothing as this could remove 80% of the contaminant (they should not remove clothing over their heads but cut them off instead)
- **Remove** the contaminant using a dry absorbent material to brush it off or soak it up. Find a water source and rinse it off if the skin is itching or burning

Clinical decontamination

The process where contaminated casualties are treated individually by trained health care professionals using purpose-designed decontamination equipment to deliver the 'rinse, wipe, rinse' method of decontamination.

Interim decontamination

The use of standard equipment to provide a planned and structured decontamination process prior to the availability of purpose-designed decontamination equipment.

Improvised decontamination

The use of an immediately available method of decontamination prior to the use of specialist resources.

Mass decontamination

A planned and structured procedure using purpose-designed decontamination equipment, where there are large numbers of casualties.

Command and control of the decontamination process

A decontamination incident warrants the inclusion of additional roles (Figure 19.2).

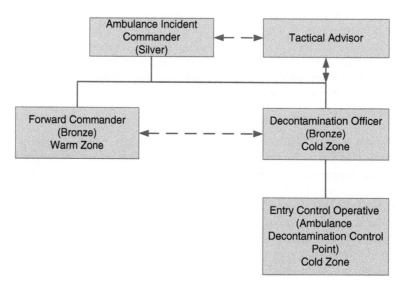

Figure 19.2 The decontamination command structure

A Forward Commander (Decontamination Officer), fully trained in decontamination procedures, should be appointed, whose sole responsibility is to oversee the decontamination process and ensure that correct procedures are adopted throughout. The prime responsibility of the Decontamination Officer is the safety of decontamination staff.

The Decontamination Officer should be located in the cold zone and will be supported by an Entry Control Operative who will manage the Entry Control Board, detailing individuals' names, roles and time of entry into the contaminated area.

Primary triage should be carried out by responders wearing chemical protective equipment. This role should be supported by a primary treatment team who can administer life-saving care, including antidotes, as required.

19.6 Summary

- The ambulance service has the lead responsibility for triage, decontamination and treatment of contaminated casualties
- The fire service usually manages the area within the inner cordon while the police are responsible for overall coordination of the response
- The inner cordon encompasses the hot and warm zones
- The hot zone includes the area directly contaminated by the release
- The warm zone is the area contaminated by the movement of vehicles and/or people
- The initial response should be REMOVE, REMOVE, REMOVE

CHAPTER 20
Incidents involving large numbers of children

Learning outcomes

After reading this chapter you will be able to:
- Describe how preparation for an incident involving large numbers of children is different
- Discuss how are children triaged at a major incident
- Discuss challenges in the treatment of children at major incidents

20.1 Introduction

For many individuals in the health service, the prospect of dealing with a major incident resulting in large numbers of injured children is daunting. For this reason, these incidents are special. Such incidents do occur both in the UK and abroad (Table 20.1). Major incidents can arise from a variety of causes and children are not excluded from any particular type of incident.

Table 20.1 Major incidents known to have involved significant numbers of children

Major incident	Year	Total number of casualties	Number of paediatric casualties
Martinez coach crash, USA	1975	51	50
Mass lightning strike, USA	1977	47	47
Bologna bombing, Italy	1980	291	27
M5 coach crash, UK	1983	31	27
Chemical gas leak, Arizona, USA	1987	>67	67
Enniskillin bombing, Northern Ireland	1987	65	6
Three Rivers regatta accident, USA	1990	24	16
Dimmocks Cote train crash, UK	1992	45	12
Avianca plane disaster, USA	1993	92	22
York coach crash, UK	1994	41	40
Abbeyhill junction train crash, UK	1994	47	10
Oklahoma bombing, USA	1995	759	61
Manchester bombing, UK	1996	217	30
Dunblane mass shooting, UK	1996	30	28
Beslan siege, Russia	2004	>700	>335
Utoeya Island shooting, Norway	2011	69	30
Manchester Arena bombing, UK	2017	162	89

Major Incident Medical Management and Support: The Practical Approach at the Scene, Fourth Edition.
Edited by Tony Gleeson and Kevin Mackway-Jones.
© 2023 John Wiley & Sons Ltd. Published 2023 by John Wiley & Sons Ltd.

Difficulties in the management of children during a major incident have been documented at all stages of the incident response. In the pre-hospital phase, problems have been identified in determining triage and transport priorities and in obtaining adequate amounts of paediatric equipment. Few hospitals are staffed or equipped to deal with any more than a few seriously ill or injured children, with well-documented shortages of paediatric surgical and intensive care unit beds. Specialist services for children are geographically scattered and confined to specialist hospitals which are not always co-located with emergency departments. This distribution of specialist services may make it difficult to get children to specialist centres during a major incident.

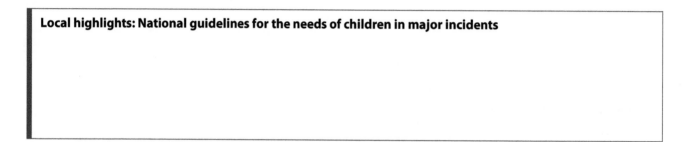

Local highlights: National guidelines for the needs of children in major incidents

20.2 Preparation

Planning

An incident involving a large number of children may require a regional or multi-regional response. Health authorities and the ambulance service should ensure that they have adequate plans for the management of children in major incidents. Mechanisms for alerting and supporting specialist centres must be in place. Close liaison between pre-hospital, receiving hospital and specialist children's services must take place.

Equipment

As mentioned above, children are involved in many major incidents and equipment is widely available, therefore the ambulance service should ensure that they have adequate supplies of paediatric equipment on their major incident support vehicles. Specific arrangements may be required to ensure the supplementation of hospital supplies from specialist children's hospitals.

In the UK there is a national reserve stock of equipment held by the ambulance service; 20% of the equipment is for children. This can be used locally, regionally and nationally as required.

Training

It is important that children take part in all major incident practices where they might in reality be present and that the age of the children matches that which might be present in a real incident. Children can provide very useful feedback about matters not immediately obvious to adults.

20.3 Medical support

Triage

The standard triage sieve and triage sort are based on adult physiological values. As children have higher pulse rates, higher respiratory rates and lower blood pressures (Table 20.2) they will usually be over-triaged if these are used. The sieve, as discussed in Chapter 15, has been modified to accommodate this.

In incidents involving small numbers of children, this is unlikely to be a significant problem as there may be practical and humanitarian reasons to remove children from the scene at an early stage. However, in incidents involving large numbers of children, systematic over-triage may adversely affect the overall response as no effective prioritisation will occur. To compensate for this, a paediatric triage tape has been developed that modifies the triage sieve according to children's normal physiological variables (Figure 20.1).

Table 20.2 Normal physiological values for children

Age (years)	Respiratory rate (breaths/min)	Pulse rate (beats/min)
<1	30–40	110–160
1–2	25–35	100–150
2–5	25–30	95–140
5–12	20–25	80–120
>12	15–20	60–100

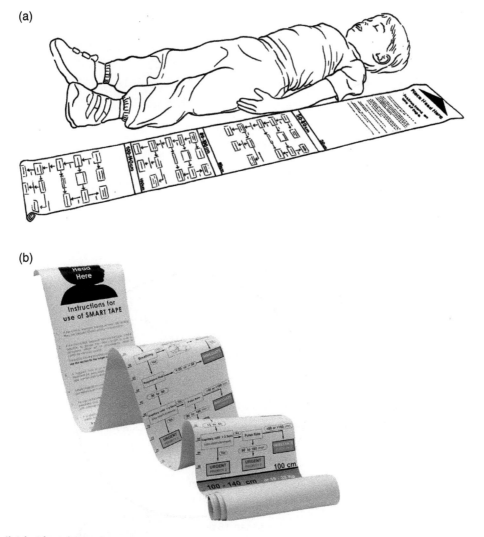

Figure 20.1 Paediatric triage tape.
Reproduced with permission of TSG Associates LLP

The paediatric triage tape is based on the approximate length to weight correlation for children aged 1–10 years. It is similar to the Broselow tape used in children but is limited to triage only. A series of modified triage sieve algorithms have been produced using the normal ranges of vital signs. These algorithms are arranged in boxes on a linear waterproof tape that is laid next to the child. Where the child's heel touches the tape indicates the algorithm to be used for that length of child.

This system means that triage officers can more accurately assess the physiological derangement in children, and in addition there is no need to remember all the variables as they are written on the tape. On occasion, the position of the child may make it impossible to use the tape but the algorithms can still be used based on age (Figures 20.2, 20.3 and 20.4).

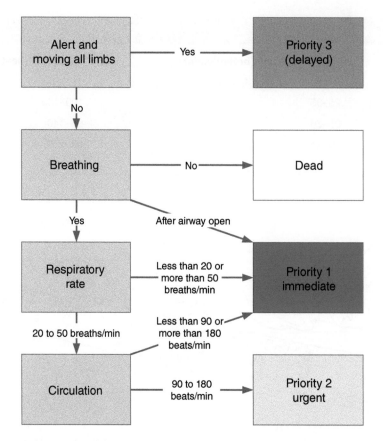

Figure 20.2 Paediatric sieve, 50–80 cm or 3–10 kg

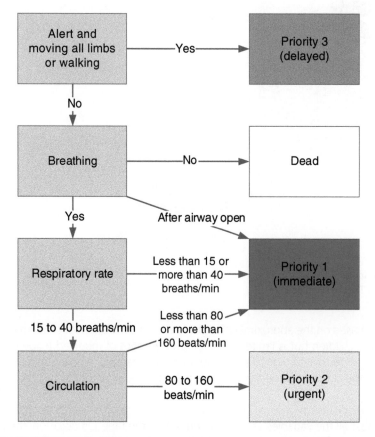

Figure 20.3 Paediatric sieve, 80–100 cm or 11–18 kg

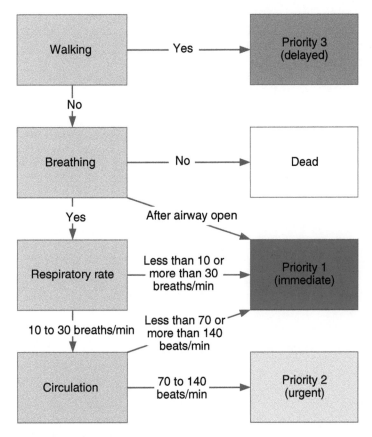

Figure 20.4 Paediatric sieve, 100–140 cm or 19–32 kg

There is no validated means to triage sort children. In incidents involving small numbers of children then they can be over-triaged using the sort mechanism for adults. This has the advantage of progressing children through the scene more quickly. However, the lack of a sort mechanism can produce problems when large numbers of children are involved in an incident as the adult sort triage will not differentiate the children appropriately. Clinical acumen may be required to decide priorities for treatment and transport.

Treatment

Pre-hospital responders may find dealing with children difficult. In particular, they may be unfamiliar with the normal physiological and psychological responses of children to illness or injury.

A number of other issues may complicate the response:

- *Scene safety*: Rescuers are willing to take greater risks when a child is involved. Emotions cloud judgement – so every precaution should be taken to prevent unnecessary risk taking
- *Families*: Major incidents may involve more than one family member. Ideally members of the same family should be kept together, but this may not always be possible if a patient's injuries require specialist care
- *Media*: There will be a high level of media interest at an incident involving children

Definitive care

It is highly likely that in an incident involving large numbers of children, emergency services may require additional help from regional services such as paediatric intensive care units and paediatric surgical units. Planners must liaise with these groups to agree a method for support during an incident.

Recovery phase

Incidents involving children are more likely to result in psychological morbidity for the rescuers. All people involved in the response must be alert to such problems in themselves and their colleagues.

20.4 Summary

- Children are often involved in major incidents
- Planning, equipment provision and training should reflect this
- The triage sieve can be modified to better reflect the physiology of younger children

CHAPTER 21
Incidents involving multiple casualties with burns

Learning outcomes

After reading this chapter you will be able to:
- Discuss the factors that influence the management of burns injuries in a major incident
- Describe the role of the burns specialist advice/specialist care teams
- Define the role of the National Burns Bed Bureau

21.1 Introduction

The initial resuscitation of a casualty involved in a major incident and sustaining a burn injury should follow the standard ABC approach. Whilst the burns are often very evident, the potential for other injuries should not be overlooked.

Initially, casualties with burns may appear to be less physiologically injured than they actually are. The potential for gradual loss of the airway is well recognised, but the delay in assessment or failure to correctly assess the burn surface area (leading to delayed and inadequate fluid resuscitation) can also significantly impair the quality of care. The initial management of significantly burned patients should follow the major trauma pathway unless specific pathways are in place for their management locally.

The provision of pre-hospital care at scene and transit to the emergency department is primarily the responsibility of the ambulance service – this can be enhanced by Medical Emergency Response Incident Teams (MERIT), Helicopter Emergency Medical Services (HEMS) and Immediate Care Doctors.

Only in very unusual circumstances would burn specialists be asked to deliver care at the scene of a burn major incident or emergency. If this were required, it is envisaged that burn specialists would assist as members of a MERIT team or similar rather than as members of free-standing burn specialist teams. Triage of patients should be undertaken in accordance with locally agreed protocols and procedures. It is recommended that burn-injured patients be referred to the appropriate local burn service at the first available opportunity.

Once the acute phase of care is complete and resuscitation well underway, burn-injured patients have a very prolonged post-acute period of care that can run to weeks or even months. The multidisciplinary nature of this, involving specialist nursing, physiotherapy, psychology and even social care, is very time and resource intensive.

Major Incident Medical Management and Support: The Practical Approach at the Scene, Fourth Edition.
Edited by Tony Gleeson and Kevin Mackway-Jones.
© 2023 John Wiley & Sons Ltd. Published 2023 by John Wiley & Sons Ltd.

21.2 Capacity

The total number of burns units and dedicated burns beds is always very limited. In most domains, it would not require a particularly large number of cases to overwhelm a single unit's capacity.

In response, National Burns Bed Bureaus (NBBBs) have been established in many countries to maintain a regularly updated log of burns bed availability and provide a network of burn care facilities. The intention is that patients with significant burns injuries can be transferred across the country to a dedicated bed as quickly as possible, potentially direct from the scene of an incident.

In the UK, the National Burns Major Incident Plan identifies various burn care networks and stratifies the levels of care for burn-injured patients and designates:

- Burn centres – that have a high level of critical care immediate theatre access
- Burn units – that have the ability to deal with moderate level injury complexity
- Burn facilities – that have a standard plastic surgical ward that can deal with non-complex injuries

While the scale of the incident is being established, no patients will be moved. Once the scale is known a distribution plan for the casualties requiring specialist care will be made.

21.3 Burns specialist advice team/burns specialist care team

All trauma centres/units should be able to provision the initial resuscitation of burns patients. Early liaison with specialist burns teams is important.

An off-site burns specialist advice team (BSAT), consisting of an experienced burns surgery consultant and a senior burns nurse, will provide advice to other clinicians. A burns specialist care team (BSCT) also consisting of an experienced burns surgery resident or consultant and senior burns nurses would provide direct patient care.

It may be possible for the coordinating unit to deploy more than one team but adjacent burns units may need to make one or more BSCTs available to assist the primary unit.

Once a fully informed burns casualty profile has been determined, a distribution plan can be created. The BSATs may then be able to act as retrieval teams to bring the patients back to their units.

21.4 Patient dispersal

Emergency departments typically care for minor burns injuries as a routine. Those patients, who have injuries that do not pass the threshold requiring fluid resuscitation or not involving danger areas such as hands, feet or perineum, can be managed at the local hospital.

At the other end of the spectrum, there are patients who are so severely burned that palliative care is the only reasonable option in a major burns incident. The 'burn index' (the sum of the patient's age and their percentage burn) can be used to identify patients who are likely to have a poor outcome and meet this decision threshold. Those with an index >100 might be managed expectantly and transfer to a burns unit might not be appropriate. A poor pre-morbid state and involvement of the airway in the burn are also markers of poor progress but are difficult to quantify.

Patients with significant burns should be managed in a unit with the specialist skills to care for them. This may require long-distance transfers. It is possible that transfer to burns units across international borders may be needed.

21.5 Summary

- Burns-injured casualties need specialist assessment and management
- The capacity of a burns unit is very limited and patient dispersal is likely to be very wide
- Burns specialist care teams should attend the receiving emergency departments, as determined by the local coordinating burns centre, to assist with assessment and management of burn-injured patients, providing an expert assessment to inform the coordinating unit
- Minor burns patients are likely to be managed locally. Severely burned patients who are unlikely to survive may be managed palliatively at the original receiving facility

CHAPTER 22
Mass gatherings

Learning outcomes

After reading this chapter you will be able to:
- Define a mass gathering
- Describe how pre-planning of mass gatherings contributes to the major incident response

---

22.1 Introduction

Mass gatherings present their own unique set of problems – fortunately, with adequate planning, most can be anticipated. The planned response should follow a generic approach; in addition, specific risks should be identified and planned for. If an incident occurs at a pre-planned mass gathering event, the response is slightly different to that of an unplanned event, in that the basic major incident management structure is often in place prior to the incident. Consequently, senior decision makers are present at the very early stages of the incident to coordinate the response. The pre-event planning will have identified the potential risks, have pre-allocated areas for tactical control officers, casualty clearing and body holding and will normally have pre-identified an ambulance parking area and 'blue routes' to and from the event for major incident vehicles

---

> **Key point**
>
> A mass gathering incident can be regarded as a planned potential major incident.

22.2 What is a mass gathering?

Mass gatherings are defined differently around the world. In the UK and the USA, a crowd of more than one thousand people is regarded as a mass gathering. The vast majority of events involving this number of people are anticipated and organised in advance and a number of important decisions can be made in advance (Figure 22.1). A small number of gatherings of this size may occur without pre-planning. The response to these should follow generic principles.

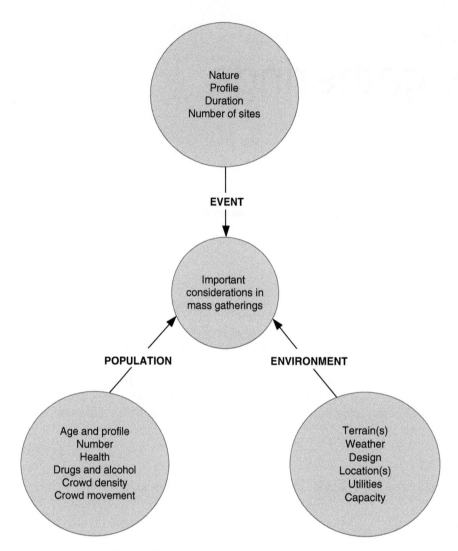

Figure 22.1 Risk factors to be considered when planning mass gathering events

The event

Stadium-based sporting events can attract large numbers of people to relatively small areas, while in other sporting events the spectators can be dispersed more widely. Religious events can attract huge numbers to a site, for example, the Hajj attracts 2 million pilgrims to Mecca on an annual basis. Political demonstrations are not uncommon and frequently occur in large cities and involve large numbers of people.

Many mass gathering events only last for hours while others (for example music festivals, sporting competitions) take place over much longer periods (days or weeks).

With increasing security at obvious terrorist targets, attacks on softer targets and iconic venues have become more likely.

The environment

Outdoor events are influenced by the weather, which will vary considerably by season and from one region of the world to another.

The movement of people at a mass gathering event increases the chance of injuries occurring. The high-risk times are at the start, the interval and the end, when large numbers of people move simultaneously. Events where people are seated are easier to plan and control as the number of seats dictates the crowd capacity. The design of modern stadia is such that the size of groups is controlled. Venue design can give rise to difficulties of access for emergency services.

The population

An important factor in determining the predicted medical need is the nature of the population attending the event. Events attract different populations, for example young adults at music festivals (and alcohol consumption may be high) or a large number of children at some football matches.

22.3 Preparation and planning

Any organising body of a mass gathering needs to ensure that local and national guidelines are consulted and followed. In the UK, the 'Green Guide' provides guidance on the accommodation and management of crowds within sports grounds. The 'Purple Guide' provides tools and guidance for the management of outdoor events such as pop concerts and festivals.

Local highlights: Mass gatherings – local and national guidelines

---

It is, of course, not possible to anticipate every eventuality when planning for mass gatherings. Where specific risks are identified, modifications to the plan can be made. Any proposed response should involve parties with knowledge of the local environment and those with experience in previous and similar events. Any planned response to an incident should use existing emergency service hierarchies, and major incident roles must be allocated to people with relevant experience and training. The allocation of roles should take place at a briefing before the event starts so that personnel can familiarise themselves with their roles before spectators arrive. Senior members of each emergency service in attendance should always be in communication during the event.

22.4 Training

Having staff in place prior to a mass gathering event is of little value unless they are competent to deal with likely eventualities. On-site exercises are useful to ensure a coordinated response. Paper and table-top exercises will help to reinforce this and can be used to validate event plans.

22.5 Summary

- A significant amount of planning is required to prepare for a major incident response at a mass gathering event. This amount of planning may also be dictated by legislation
- Unlike other major incident responses, considerable thought can be given to the scene set-up and response prior to the event
- The management structure at a mass gathering event is frequently in place prior to the event, helping to ensure a rapid response to any incident that occurs

CHAPTER 23
Natural disasters

Learning outcomes

After reading this chapter you will be able to:
- Describe natural disasters
- List common types of natural disaster
- Discuss the human impact on the frequency and severity of natural disasters
- Describe why there is a need for planning for natural disaster
- Discuss natural disaster mitigation techniques

23.1 Introduction

Natural disasters are often devastating and have caused massive loss of life, an inestimable number of injuries and rendered millions homeless over recorded time. They can be classified into different types (Table 23.1).

Table 23.1 Classification of natural disasters

Geological	Meteorological	Biological
Earthquake	Cyclone, hurricane and typhoon	Flu and other pandemics
Tsunami	Floods	Famine
Volcano	Fires	Pests
Landslide and avalanches	Heatwaves	

In this chapter, the mechanism for each type of natural disaster is discussed, together with mitigation and response as appropriate.

The number of natural disasters is likely to increase as man's effect on nature increases. There is always the threat that a single natural disaster may have the potential to threaten humankind. Some texts have termed this a 'mega-disaster'. Evidence of this type of disaster exists – for example the ending of the Cretaceous period (and the disappearance of the dinosaurs amongst most of the rest of the planet's life forms) 65 million years ago.

23.2 Geological disasters

Earthquakes

Earthquakes have caused enormous casualties over time as shown in Table 23.2.

Relief expertise is growing rapidly. Significant advances include the caching of large supplies of basic shelters, tents and bedding. Urban search and rescue (USAR) teams with specific training and equipment are becoming expert in finding and retrieving live victims from rubble many days after an earthquake.

Major Incident Medical Management and Support: The Practical Approach at the Scene, Fourth Edition.
Edited by Tony Gleeson and Kevin Mackway-Jones.
© 2023 John Wiley & Sons Ltd. Published 2023 by John Wiley & Sons Ltd.

Tsunamis

Tsunamis (from the Japanese words for harbour (*tsu*) and wave (*nami*)) are large waves created by sudden movements in the seabed, usually by earthquakes, volcanoes (for example Krakatau, Indonesia, 1883), landslides and meteorite ember strikes. The devastating tsunami on 26 December 2004, affected northern Sumatra/Aceh, Malaysia, Thailand, Myanmar, Sri Lanka and the Maldives, and beaches as far away as Madagascar and East Africa. Estimates put the final death toll at over 300 000.

Mitigation techniques for tsunamis include an early warning system together with systems of alerts and sirens in towns and villages across vulnerable regions. Major projects are now underway to reforest mangrove tidal plains, particularly around towns and cities.

Volcanoes

Volcanic eruptions can range from the gentle to the explosive and catastrophic. Several large eruptions have produced massive local loss of life, such as Tamboro, Sumbawa, Indonesia in 1815, killing 92 000.

Mitigation techniques for volcanic eruption depend on seismic activity and motion sensors, satellite imagery and thermal monitoring to alert scientists of impending eruption.

Landslides/avalanches

Landslides are mass movements of soil/mud and rock, often triggered by heavy rain, an earthquake or volcanic eruption. One example is the landslide of mining waste that occurred in Aberfan, Wales, in 1966, burying 144 people including 116 school children.

Mitigation planning for all forms of avalanche and landslide centre around building controls, particularly in steep terrain with high precipitation (rain or snow). Building codes and deflective walls and roofs around towns and roads contribute to safety. Reforestation has helped prevent snow and soil/mud avalanches across the globe. Early warnings occur in some regions and can allow high-risk areas to be evacuated.

Table 23.2 Sites, dates and deaths from earthquakes

Site	Date	Deaths/injuries
Shaanxi, China	1556	830 000 dead
Lisbon, Portugal	1755	60 000–100 000 dead
Izmit, Turkey	1999	17 100 dead
Bam, Iran	2003	31 000 dead
Kashmir, northern Pakistan	2005	90 000 dead, 110 000 injured
Yogyakarta, Indonesia	2006	6200 dead, 46 000 injured
Shaanxi, China	2008	65 000 dead
Earthquake and tsunami, Tohoku, Japan	2011	15 894 dead, 6152 injured Subsequent nuclear accident
Bridge collapse, Genoa, Italy	2018	43 dead, over 15 injured Bridge collapse after heavy rain

23.3 Meteorological disasters

Hurricanes/tropical cyclones/typhoons

These are caused by tropical depressions of sufficient intensity to produce sustained wind speeds of greater than 63 km/h. These storms have different names according to their location, being called tropical cyclones in the Indian, South Pacific or South Atlantic Oceans, typhoons in the rest of Asia and hurricanes in the Americas and Caribbean. They require a sea surface temperature in excess of 27°C (81°F) and, as sea temperatures rise, scientists believe the rate, range and ferocity of these storms will increase. Wind speeds govern the classification number of each storm.

Tropical storms occur in some of the poorest and most heavily populated areas of the world. The category 4 cyclone, Nargis, hit Myanmar in May 2008. The actual casualty number is still uncertain, but ranges from 100 000 to 300 000. As well as destructive winds and heavy rains with flooding, cyclones can cause storm surges as strong winds push sea water toward the coast. Hurricane Katrina in August 2008, with category 3 winds, caused some of the damage but it was the 8–10-metre (27–34-foot) storm surge that swamped the New Orleans levee sea defences, covered 80% of the city and destroyed some surrounding towns. Official casualties are recorded at 1836 dead and 705 missing.

Mitigation planning takes the form of early warning systems managed by weather bureaus and engineering design to protect low-lying areas like New Orleans. Public education on the need for personal cyclone shelters and emergency kits, including food for several days, can be broadcast before and during each cyclone season.

Cyclone and hurricane tracking allows governments to assess the threat and need for evacuation several days before they hit land. All these mitigation techniques have been implemented in developed nations with resources, but in areas of Bangladesh, India and the Caribbean, no such warning systems or building codes occur and the threat of tropical cyclones remains extreme.

Floods

Flooding is the inundation of land by large amounts of water (Table 23.3) and can be a consequence of excessive precipitation or from storm surges (see previous section).

Table 23.3 Sites, dates and deaths from floods

Site	Date	Deaths/injuries
Galveston, Texas, USA	1900	8000 dead
Yangtze, China	1931	400 000 dead
Bangladesh	1974	28 700 dead
Vargas, Venezuela	1999	20 000 dead
North India	2013	5700 dead
Henan, China	2021	300 dead

Fires

Wildfires, in grass or forest, can spread uncontrollably and pose a significant threat to human settlement and property (Table 23.4). They have been occurring with increasing frequency, which has been attributed to climate change. Fires in urban environments can also become uncontrolled, despite fire 'watches' and firefighting services. After the devastating Tokyo earthquake of 1923, a fire killed thousands of the 143 000 casualties. Wildfires in Canberra, Australia in 2003 and in California in 2005 have caused significant damage to property and vegetation, and some loss of life.

Control and mitigation techniques for wildfires include back burning and ensuring fuel load (e.g. dry, dead vegetation) is kept under control before hot, dry conditions arrive, particularly around rural–urban interfaces. Mitigation techniques in urban environments include smoke detectors, fire extinguishing systems and an effective firefighting service in almost every town and city in the world.

Table 23.4 Sites, dates and deaths from wildfires

Site	Date	Deaths/injuries
Victoria, Australia (Black Saturday Bushfires)	2009	173 dead
Yarnell, Arizona, USA	2013	19 dead
Attica, Greece	2018	100 dead, 170 injured
California, USA	2020	33 dead, 37 injured

Heatwaves

Heatwaves are defined as prolonged periods of excessively hot weather. There is no universally agreed temperature definition, rather it depends on exceeding the normal ambient temperature scales for the area, often for several days in succession. In the USA, heatwaves kill more than hurricanes, tornadoes, lightning and floods combined. The heatwave of New York in 1980 killed up to 1600 people, whilst the European heatwave of August 2003 is estimated to have caused 35 000 deaths.

The very young and old are particularly at risk. Cities display a phenomenon known as the 'urban heat island' due to heat absorption by fixed structures like roads and buildings. Mitigation of this phenomenon with parks and heat-dissipating buildings have recently become part of urban planning. Avoidance of power failures contributes to lives saved. Emergency 'cooling centres' may help, particularly for the elderly who may not be able to afford air-conditioning.

Flu and pandemics

In December 2019, the emergence of Covid-19 coronavirus in Wuhan Provence, China heralded a worldwide pandemic over the following months as the coronavirus spread outside China to over 110 countries worldwide. On 11 March 2020, a pandemic was declared by the World Health Organization. Despite attempts to halt the spread, the numbers of affected individuals continued to increase. Mitigation of the spread of the virus was attempted by governments around the world which responded with lockdowns and restrictions on populations to reduce contact and spread of the illness. Early sequencing of the genome was also performed to aid the development and trials of vaccines to counter it. It took until December 2020 for a vaccine to be approved for use in the general population, with the UK being the first country worldwide to approve use of Pfizer/BioNTech Covid-19 vaccination. The gradual slow but existential spread of the virus is often referred to as a 'rising tide' in major incident terms.

Famine

A famine occurs when there is a widespread scarcity of food and despite efforts to prevent famines occurring, they still do affect many parts of the world, especially sub-Saharan Africa. The causes of such food shortages can be multifactorial including poor governance, failure of crops (environmental factors), war, inflation and imbalances in population. The numbers of people dying from malnutrition and famine has dropped considerably from the late twentieth century, through the introduction of mitigation factors such as government support, charitable agencies, global partnerships and the development of food stores to support populations affected.

Pests

Spread of illness and pandemics from pests are not seen very often in the world these days. The Black Death or bubonic plague pandemic that occurred in the 1300s, affecting Europe and Asia, was caused by a bacteria *Yersinia pestis*, spread by fleas which picked up the bacteria from infected rats. It caused the death of 20 million people in Europe. Mitigation of spread in modern days is through increased hygiene and the introduction of bio-security measures by countries.

23.4 Summary

- Natural disasters have befallen humankind since records began. Climate change and an increasing world population ensure that numbers will rise
- Mitigation of natural disasters, particularly in resource-rich nations, has advanced significantly
- Planning, in the form of engineering and building codes, early warning systems and evacuation, public education and stockpiling of equipment, has already proven effective
- Mitigation techniques and planning is far cheaper and more effective in the long term than reaction and rebuilding after a natural disaster
- Planning locally relevant and effective projects to mitigate local threats may prove a more cost-effective method of aid from rich to poor nations than disaster relief teams once a catastrophe has occurred
- Response needs to be proportionate to need

CHAPTER 24
Uncompensated major incidents

Learning outcomes

After reading this chapter you will be able to:
- Describe an uncompensated major incident
- Discuss the factors that contribute to making an incident uncompensated
- Describe how treatment aims may be changed during an uncompensated major incident

---

24.1 Introduction

An uncompensated incident occurs when the medical resources mobilised in response to a major incident are inadequate to deal with the number of casualties, that is, 'load exceeds capacity'. Most uncompensated major incidents are a result of *natural* events such as floods or earthquakes, in which case these incidents are also *compound*. Occasionally, *man-made* incidents can be of such magnitude that the casualty load exceeds the capacity of the health system. An example of an uncompensated man-made incident was that in Bhopal, India on 3 December 1984 when a valve on a tank of methyl isocyanate burst, releasing a toxic cloud that killed an estimated 8000 people and left 170 000 disfigured or disabled.

Key point

In an uncompensated incident the load of live casualties is greater than the capacity of the system.

The capacity of a health system to respond to the patient load in a major incident varies between countries and between regions within a country. A bomb blast leaving 200 live casualties in the middle of a large western city is likely to be a compensated major incident, whereas the same event in a city in the developing world is likely to be uncompensated. Similarly, a major incident involving 20 live casualties in a remote rural area is likely to remain an uncompensated incident for many hours, resulting in potential increased morbidity and mortality. A major incident may move from being initially uncompensated to become compensated as more resources are mobilised to treat casualties.

Key point

A major incident may move from being initially uncompensated to become compensated as more resources are mobilised to treat casualties.

Major Incident Medical Management and Support: The Practical Approach at the Scene, Fourth Edition.
Edited by Tony Gleeson and Kevin Mackway-Jones.
© 2023 John Wiley & Sons Ltd. Published 2023 by John Wiley & Sons Ltd.

24.2 Factors contributing to an incident being uncompensated

For a given live casualty load, it is the capacity of the health system *during the major incident response* that determines whether the incident will be compensated or uncompensated. If there is a lack of *surge capacity planning*, a *lack of resources* or *compounding factors* in the incident the health capacity will be diminished and the incident is more likely to be uncompensated.

Surge capacity planning

Historically, major incident planning evolved in response to deficiencies identified when a major incident had recently occurred. Increasingly, more strategic planning is a funded priority; this involves a risk assessment (at local, regional and national levels) and the development of integrated multiagency plans to meet the needs of potential incidents. Planning for major incidents has become a political priority in many parts of the world due to recent 'spectacular' terrorist incidents.

Planning for major incidents can greatly enhance available resources at the time of an incident by focusing local resource to the major incident, using disaster stockpiles, using other agency's resources and using novel resources that are not part of day-to-day operations. For larger incidents, regional, national and even international resources may need to be mobilised. Written and practiced plans are essential, as are negotiated interagency agreements so that at the time of the response all parties are aware of their roles and responsibilities. Predetermined casualty capability arrangements are a part of mass casualty planning and will assist with the dispersal of casualties within an existing health care system.

Major incident planning creates 'surge capacity' in the system, which may be many times the normal day-to-day operational capacity (Box 24.1). In the modern health environment, where hospitals often run at 90–100% bed occupancy and use 'just in time' supplies, there is very little 'slack' in the system to face the casualty load of a major incident.

Box 24.1 Creating surge capacity in the health system

Command and control	• Intra- and interagency agreements and written protocols • Succession planning built into the command structure so that there is a wide pool to call upon rather than just a few individuals
Communications	• Deploying a separate 'medical' radio net or having arrangements and equipment to link into the ambulance radio net • Deploying satellite phones • Having protected mobile phone handsets if the cellular network is shut down in response to a terrorist event
Treatment	• Equipment/consumables: disaster stockpiles or 'pods' • Bed spaces: rapid discharge rounds; buying step-down beds, e.g. in local hotels; sharing load amongst local and regional hospitals; sharing specialist unit (e.g. burns unit, intensive care unit) workload through a national network • International transfers for specialist services • Staffing: importing regional staff to fill rosters; using medical students as 'runners'; using GPs and retired medical practitioners
Transport	• Using ambulances from the region • Mutual aid arrangements with adjoining regions • Using coaches/buses from commercial companies • Using military assets for transport

Without effective planning, even small incidents, apparently within the theoretical capacity of the local health system, can become uncompensated because resources are not available in the right place at the right time. The larger the casualty load, the greater the need for mobilisation of resources and the greater the need for effective planning at every level.

Fixed resources

Resources (for example hospital beds, operating theatres, staff, ambulances, helicopters, communications, roads, police service, fire service) are largely fixed in a particular area. The resources present are determined by wealth and population.

Thus, for a given live casualty load, poorer nations and remote regions are more likely to experience an uncompensated major incident.

Compounding factors

A compound incident is one where the infrastructure involved in the major incident response is damaged at the time of the response. Compounding factors remove resources and disrupt plans (i.e. diminish the capacity of the health system to respond to the major incident) and so increase the chance of the load exceeding capacity. Compounding factors in an incident can be isolated to one part of the system or generalised and affect all or most of the infrastructure in a community. They are summarised in Table 24.1.

Table 24.1 Compounding factors in a major incident

Compounding factors	Examples
Transport damage	Flood, earthquake, severe weather (aircraft cannot fly), terrorism target
Hospital damage	Flood, earthquake, severe weather (e.g. cyclones), power failure to hospital with no back-up supply, terrorism target
Communication damage	Overload of a mobile phone net by a worried population, equipment failure, weather conditions preventing satellite phone use, terrorism target
Widespread infrastructure damage	Natural disaster, war, civil unrest, massive man-made incident

24.3 Case studies

Case study 1 Remote major incident: Australian outback 2008

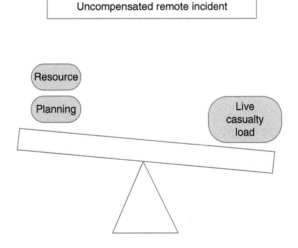

A single vehicle rollover in the Australian outback at night, on a dirt road 300 km from the nearest hospital, 10 km from the nearest airstrip and 30 km from the only local health facility. Local resources consisted of a remote clinic with one nurse, one health worker, one four-wheel drive ambulance, one satellite phone and some medical supplies. Additionally, there was one policeman and a police vehicle. The nurse used the satellite phone to call the retrieval service coordinator about 2 hours after the crash and the call was escalated to the duty emergency physician. The satellite phone reception was intermittent due to cloud cover but eventually the transmitted information indicated that 17 people were travelling in the vehicle, one was dead (an infant), one was unconscious and 'lots' had severe injuries. On this information a local major incident was declared and two fixed wing aircraft (each with a two-stretcher capacity), two retrieval doctors, two nurses and an aerial retrieval major incident cache was dispatched along with a road ambulance with a paramedic crew. Hospital staff were put on standby. The first medical team arrived at the scene about 4 hours after the crash. Prior to the arrival of the medical teams some patients were spinally immobilised but collars had run out, most patients had had analgesia, a hypotensive patient had used up all the available crystalloid and splints had been made from branches of wood. The unconscious patient was left in the recovery position and a decision made to concentrate on the other casualties. The initial responders not only had to tend to the injured but also had to switch on the runway lights and ferry the arriving medical teams and the patients to and from the aircraft (each round trip from the scene taking an hour). The initial responders also knew all the casualties personally and some were family members. Following arrival of the medical teams, the injured underwent a MIMMS sort. One casualty was ventilated at-scene (subdural), one had an O negative transfusion (splenic laceration and pelvic fracture) and all patients had analgesia and first aid (six of the patients had hip dislocations). A satellite phone link was re-established enabling a full injury and time of arrival list to be transmitted. This resulted in the receiving hospital being able to de-escalate its response so that staff were not unnecessarily fatigued.

Learning points

The incident was initially uncompensated. The minor compounding factor of poor satellite communications did not hamper the response. Treatment aims were altered for the unconscious patient due to lack of resources. The incident became compensated with the arrival on-scene of additional resources.

Case study 2 Man-made major incident: Bali bombings 2002

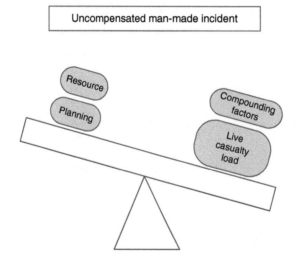

Terrorist bombs in a Bali nightclub killed 202 people, 88 of whom were Australian. Over 150 were left critically injured, many of whom were also Australian. With little idea of the casualty load due to a lack of a reliable scene assessment, the Australian government sent military Hercules aircraft with medical teams from the closest Australian hospital to retrieve the most seriously injured. Sixty-two patients with major injuries (blast and thermal injury) were retrieved to the Royal Darwin Hospital (the closest Australian hospital to Bali) – the last arriving 48 hours after the blast. Because of a lack of scene assessment, the retrieval teams did not have some equipment (for example sufficient numbers of sterile scalpels for the scores of escharotomies performed). In Bali most medical supplies had run out, and patients were found with dressings but no fluid resuscitation as this too had run out. Many were waiting to have urgent operative intervention. The Royal Darwin Hospital mobilised 1600 local staff and flew in an interstate burns team. Ambulances to transport the patients from the airport to the hospital were mobilised from throughout the region (from up to 750 km away). The injured were resuscitated (many requiring ventilation when standard burns fluid resuscitation commenced) and both 'rescue' and definitive operations were performed. The Australian Burns Plan was activated and 40 patients with severe burns were flown out to major burns centres across the continent within 48 hours of arrival in Darwin. It is estimated that 500 Australians with minor injuries made their own way back home and were treated at local hospitals in Australia.

Learning points

The major incident was uncompensated in Bali. The incident (for the Australian casualties) was compensated on arrival in Australia 1–2 days after the initial blast. Regional and national plans were activated and resources mobilised across the nation. Strategic Command was held by the Australian government.

Case study 3 Natural major incident: Hurricane Mitch, Honduras 1998

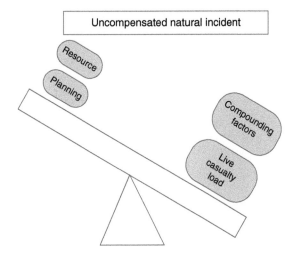

Mitch, initially a category 5 hurricane (290 km/h sustained winds with higher speed gusts) swept across Honduras, Nicaragua, El Salvador, Guatemala and Belize in October 1998. It caused an estimated 10 000 fatalities with possibly a further 10 000 missing. Hardest hit was Honduras where floods and mudslides destroyed 25 towns, 70% of the nation's crops and most roads and bridges. Hundreds of thousands of people were displaced with many still unable to return to their homes over a decade later. It is estimated that rebuilding will take a further 10 years to reach the infrastructure levels present in 1998, and that the hurricane has delayed economic development by 40–50 years. In that time there may be another natural disaster.

Learning points

This was a natural major incident that deserves the term 'catastrophe'. This compound incident, which destroyed infrastructure across many nations, never became compensated in terms of treatment for the injured and it is affecting people's lives a decade later and will do so for many years to come.

24.4 Responses to uncompensated incidents: altered treatment aims

There is always a time after the 'big bang' of a major incident when little appears to be happening for the injured. This is the time lag between the initiation of the response and the arrival of resources at the right place to help the injured. A large number of live casualties, compounding factors and lack of resources (for example remoteness) can create an incident in which there are significant delays in getting help to the casualties or getting the casualties to help – during this period the incident is uncompensated. Escalation of the incident response from local to regional to national may eventually bring enough resource to bear to make the incident compensated. This period may be hours to days, or the incident may never become compensated.

During the uncompensated phase of an incident, medical care can still be given to casualties although treatment aims may have to be altered to ensure that 'the most good is done for the most people'. At the scene and in hospitals there may be use of the 'expectant' category in patients who would, under better circumstances, be offered life-saving procedures. Operatively, the treatment strategy may, for example, change from limb reconstruction to amputation. In a viral respiratory pandemic there may be rationing of invasive ventilation support to those with the highest chance of survival (for example the young and those with no co-morbidities). The decision to alter treatment aims in any incident should be taken at the highest available level. In a remote incident this may be the most senior doctor present at-scene (if there is no communication with Strategic Command), but in most uncompensated incidents the decision should occur at Strategic Command.

Key point

During an uncompensated major incident treatment aims may have to change; the decision to do this should be made at Strategic Command.

In compound uncompensated incidents involving an entire region (for example a tsunami, earthquake or cyclone), the medical response is usually almost entirely from out of the region and can take days or weeks to arrive in sufficient mass to be effective. In these circumstances government and non-governmental agencies have to prioritise aid aims in much the same way as treatment aims are altered in smaller scale events. The priority is no longer those injured (many of whom will already be dead) but the uninjured survivors, and aid is directed to safe water, safe sanitation, food provision, shelter and communicable disease prevention (to ensure 'the most good is done for the most people').

24.5 Summary

- In an uncompensated major incident the load of live casualties is greater than the capacity of the system
- A major incident may move from being initially uncompensated to become compensated as more resources are mobilised to treat casualties
- Available resources, planning and compounding factors influence the capacity of the health system to respond to a major incident
- During an uncompensated major incident treatment aims may have to change; the decision to do this should be made at the Strategic level

CHAPTER 25
Marauding terrorist attacks

Learning outcomes

After reading this chapter you will be able to:
- Understand what a marauding terrorist attack is
- Understand how the response is a dynamic one with regular risk assessments performed to ensure staff remain safe
- Understand that staff working within the 'warm' and 'hot' zones need to be specially trained to work in those areas
- Understand what a casualty collection point is and how it integrates with the main response

---

25.1 Introduction

A marauding terrorist attack (MTA), sometimes called an active shooter or mass casualty attacker refers to an incident involving a perpetrator who has an intention to cause harm or mass murder usually in a populated or confined space, followed by, on occasions suicide. The incidence of these attacks has been seen with increased frequency over the last number of years with attacks at Nice (2016, 2020), Paris (2015) and Brussels (2016) to name but a few. Active shooter refers to the use of a firearm though this is not always the primary method of attack.

Marauding terrorist attacks are fast-moving, violent attacks where assailants move through a location aiming to find and kill or injure as many people as possible. Most deaths occur within the first few minutes, before police are able to respond.

Often there is no pattern or selection of victims, however, a particular target demographic may have been chosen by the perpetrator dependent on the ideology being utilised.

An MTA may involve:

- Bladed weapons
- Vehicle as a weapon
- Fire as a weapon
- Improvised explosive devices (IEDs)/grenades
- Firearms
- Siege (including the taking of hostages to prolong an attack or impede rescue operations)
- Chemicals in conjunction with any of the above (for example acid or alkali)

25.2 Response

The response provided by the emergency services to an MTA will be dynamic, coordinated and scalable, and may rapidly involve a significant deployment of emergency services resources.

In the event of an attack, specialist ways of working will be adopted by the emergency services and other agencies. In the UK, joint operating principles for emergency services responding to an attack have been developed setting out how the emergency services and other relevant organisations will work together. Similar operating principles are in use in other jurisdictions.

The emergency services response will be coordinated by the police. They will work with the other emergency services to assess the threat and risk and determine which areas are safe for them to enter.

Major Incident Medical Management and Support: The Practical Approach at the Scene, Fourth Edition.
Edited by Tony Gleeson and Kevin Mackway-Jones.
© 2023 John Wiley & Sons Ltd. Published 2023 by John Wiley & Sons Ltd.

The Forward Control Point (FCP) is the location where command and coordination of deployments is undertaken by a ground assigned commander and their emergency service equivalents. It is located at the boundary between the warm and cold zones. This will be jointly agreed at the time of the incident together with a Rendezvous Point (RVP) – a location to which police and emergency services personnel attending an incident may be directed. This ensures that the scene of the incident does not become inundated with resources, and personnel can be deployed in an orderly fashion. Similar to CBRNe (chemical, biological, radiological, nuclear and explosive) incidents, MTA incident sites will be zoned into hot, warm and cold in order to determine clear, hazardous and non-hazardous working areas.

25.3 Health services

In the UK, most ambulance services will have specially trained clinicians and commanders trained in the response to an MTA incident, which will be supported by traditional command structures. These resources are likely to be deployed as part of a predetermined response to any incident. Ambulance services would not deploy in the hot zone (the area of ongoing terrorist activity) and it would be usual for the deployment to the warm zone (the area adjacent to the hot area but not directly at risk) to have to be ratified by ambulance service commanders.

These are very fast-moving situations and the zoning may change very rapidly and will require an active ability to modify the health response accordingly. From a health perspective the aim is to protect any responders from potential risk of injury, whilst at the same time doing the best to help any casualty.

Ambulance services will maintain an open three-way conference call with the other emergency services in order to share information in a timely fashion and decide whether MTA resources should be deployed to an active incident.

Information shared should include:

- Confirmation of an MTA incident including a clear description of the attack methodology using plain language
- Relevant information including METHANE messages
- Location of Rendezvous Point(s) and Forward Control Point(s)
- Detail of safe approach routes
- Known or believed location and direction of movement of suspects
- Any other information which enables an effective coordinated response

A range of tactical options are available and should be considered by the Interim MTA Commanders, according to the threat and attack methodology. Recognised tactical options for the management of patients may include the modification of standard major incident triage systems in conjunction with the following casualty evacuation methods:

- **Treat and leave**
- **Treat and take**
- **Snatch rescue**

Casualties being moved from the scene are moved to a **Casualty Collection Point** at the boundary of the warm and cold zones and are then moved by a different team to the Casualty Clearing Station after triage and brief stabilising intervention. This method ensures that those trained in MTA are kept free to work in the warm zone, whilst those untrained can safely work in the cold area.

Where casualties may be a potential threat or found to be in possession of weapons, responders will immediately assess the risk and, if necessary, withdraw to a safe distance.

Receiving hospitals will be notified in the usual manner and should also consider the protection of their site during such an incident (such as implementing a lock down of their site).

25.4 Summary

- The nature of a marauding terrorist attack needs a comprehensive risk assessment and needs to be dynamic, coordinated and scalable as required
- The police will have overall control of the scene and will determine the areas where the emergency services will be able to work safely
- Staff working within the 'warm' and 'hot' zones need to be specially trained to do so

PART VII
Appendices

APPENDIX A
Psychological aspects of major incidents

A.1 Introduction

This appendix considers the psychological effects and behavioral responses of individuals, families and communities of disasters as they affect both the rescuers and the rescued. Three states will be discussed:

- Immediate effects
- Early effects
- Late effects

Psychological problems are common in the injured, in uninjured survivors and in those involved with the rescue operation following a major incident. Many more people than are physically injured can be expected to have a psychological injury. The psychological aspects will be considered here in terms of immediate, early and late problems.

> **Key point**
>
> Psychological problems are common. They occur in the injured and uninjured survivors, and the rescuers.

A.2 Immediate effects

Initially, both the injured and uninjured survivors may be anxious and upset about their injuries or about having narrowly missed being killed. These people may also be upset about friends and relatives who have been killed or injured, or who are missing.

It is less common for the rescuers to be overcome by the situation because they will be part of a coordinated and ordered response and will have seen cases of significant trauma prior to the incident. Each commander should, however, be alert to the signs of stress and fatigue in their workers and be prepared to withdraw affected individuals from the scene.

A.3 Early effects

Survivors may feel guilty at having lived through the experience when a friend or relative has died or blame themselves for their death or injury: *'If I hadn't wanted to go to Madrid that day . . .'.* Equally, those injured may feel anger and resentment towards a perceived guilty party. Such emotions should be anticipated, and help offered. Follow up can be particularly difficult. For example, an uninjured survivor of a transport disaster in one part of the country may be discharged from hospital, return home and suffer such feelings in isolation.

Major Incident Medical Management and Support: The Practical Approach at the Scene, Fourth Edition.
Edited by Tony Gleeson and Kevin Mackway-Jones.
© 2023 John Wiley & Sons Ltd. Published 2023 by John Wiley & Sons Ltd.

Health service staff who are used to dealing with suffering on an individual basis may be overwhelmed by the magnitude of the human disaster. No one is immune but junior staff can be particularly vulnerable.

Efforts must be made to offer support to all those involved using appropriate resources.

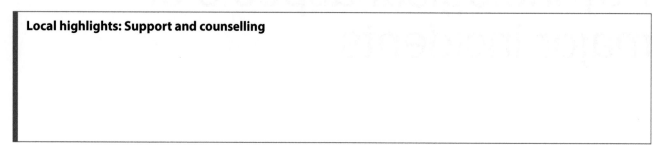

Local highlights: Support and counselling

Managers may wish to hold a short operational debrief for their staff after the 'stand down' has been announced. This will allow the opportunity to address any systems and process issues which can lead to improvement in the planning process and any future response. More importantly, there should be an opportunity for mutual support both immediately and once people have had a chance to consider the events. Open discussion should be encouraged.

Ambulance services may find it difficult to hold combined operational debriefing sessions after the event as personnel may have attended from throughout the operational area and from neighbouring ambulance services. It is imperative, therefore, to ensure that all personnel are contacted and support made available through 'peer support' and that occupational health systems are in place.

Key point

Anticipate problems and pre-empt them with adequate, early mutual support.

A.4 Late effects

Some of those exposed to an incident may suffer the symptoms of post-traumatic stress disorder (PTSD). These symptoms may persist for years after the incident. Warning signs include unpleasant flashbacks or nightmares, poor work performance, anxiety, depression or fear of associated events (such as travelling on a train after a rail incident). Formal psychiatric help may be needed.

In addition, members of staff who were not directly involved in the response to the incident may have psychological issues due to feelings of inadequacy and being unable to help. Consideration must be given to the monitoring of this group of staff as well.

Psychological support processes should follow the usual process in the country, such as existing Employee Assistance Programs and Peer Support Programs.

APPENDIX B
The media

B.1 Introduction

The media can, on occasion, be useful to major incident commanders. For example, local radio or television broadcasts can be used to reach off-duty staff or potential blood donors. More commonly, however, the media are regarded as a hindrance. It is now usual for a large number of newspaper, radio and television reporters to attend the scene of any large incident within a very short time. Initially these are likely to be local reporters, but national and international interest must be anticipated. Firm management is required, while allowing the media adequate access to report the incident.

Social media can be used as an important tool when gathering intelligence. Intelligence is information which has been confirmed. It can be used to mount a response by allowing two-way communication with our 'customers' and control rooms or commanders in order to gain information that can be potentially used to assist the response. Healthcare organisations should not ignore social media and it is advisable to consider appointing a commander to work with internal media staff to gather information and respond as needed.

B.2 At the scene

The management of the media is the responsibility of the police. The media expect to be given the opportunity to report and access to photograph, film and talk to key personnel. Unmanaged, they may contaminate the scene of crime, obstruct the emergency services and intrude upon the dignity of the injured. If over-restricted, they may resort to unethical tactics to obtain the information they need to meet their production deadlines. However, properly respected they can be managed with regular information, interviews with senior officers and photographic opportunities.

Box B.1 lists the key areas to address that will produce good media relations while maintaining control. The police services will be responsible for coordinating these; however they may request a medical spokesperson to assist them during interviews.

Box B.1 Requirements for effective media handling

- Creation of a media rendezvous point
- Restriction of access to the scene
- Provision of a Media Liaison Officer
- Consideration of the provision of a media centre
- Provision of regular information updates to coincide with television/radio bulletins
- Strict maintenance of an even-handed approach
- Provision of a public relations manager in extended incidents

Media representatives attending the scene should be given a rendezvous point which is beyond the outer cordon. This will allow control of all personnel entering the scene to be maintained. *Access* of media to the scene may be allowed and passes issued to clearly identify the individuals. It is likely that only a limited number will be given this privilege, for security and safety

Major Incident Medical Management and Support: The Practical Approach at the Scene, Fourth Edition.
Edited by Tony Gleeson and Kevin Mackway-Jones.
© 2023 John Wiley & Sons Ltd. Published 2023 by John Wiley & Sons Ltd.

reasons, and the media should be allowed to choose who their representatives will be (picking, for example, a television crew, a newspaper reporter, a radio crew and a photographer – known as a 'media pool'). It is unwise to favour particular representatives, as others will be encouraged to get the information they need by any means, regardless of whether they have to resort to unreliable eye witnesses or threaten the security of the scene. Parking space for outside broadcast units should be considered, so that access routes are not restricted by large vehicles. Rules for aerial photography must be decided upon early and emergency flying restrictions imposed if necessary. Helicopters are commonly used by the media but the resultant noise and downdraft may inhibit the work of rescuers, produce hazards from flying debris and destroy or alter forensic evidence.

The Media Liaison Officer from each of the emergency services should provide information updates at regular, specified intervals, therefore encouraging the media to wait for this information rather than searching for their own. It is important to avoid injudicious suppositions as to the cause of the incident, which cannot fully be known in the early phases of the rescue operation, and to concentrate on commenting on how the rescue is progressing.

This is aided by directing all information through one individual. The media will be offered brief interviews with emergency service commanders and this can include the Ambulance and Medical Commanders. It is wise to prepare a statement rather than allow a free question interview. Box B.2 shows the likely flow of questions and Box B.3 shows a checklist that can be used when preparing for a media interview. The Medical Commander should brief his or her staff on how to react to an approach by the media; estimates of the number of casualties or dead should not be given unless these have been confirmed.

Box B.2 Anticipated progression of questions

- What happened?
- What are the injuries/fatalities?
- What are you doing about it?
- Why did it happen?
- Who is responsible?

Box B.3 Checklist for a television interview

Before the interview

- Think of your objectives – what are the points you want to get across?
- Ask what the first question will be
- Ascertain what the 'wind up' signal is
- Check your appearance

During the interview

- Always assume you are on the air
- Look straight at the interviewer, not the camera
- Avoid jargon, swearing, lying, fidgeting and losing your cool
- Sell yourself: others will be only too ready to criticise
- Express sympathy for the injured/dead and their families
- Express admiration for the rescue workers and your own staff

After the interview

- Stand still until it is clear you are off the air
- Distribute copies of any prepared statement

A *media centre* should be considered in a large or prolonged incident; it will be the responsibility of the police and the local authorities to organise this. It may initially be in a command vehicle or a nearby building and will provide a focal point for continuing media coordination. It should contain communications equipment, an area for briefings, an area to monitor current media broadcasts and possibly accommodation for the reporters.

A *public relations manager* can contribute significantly to the smooth handling of the media and running of the media centre. Suitable individuals should be identified in the planning stages and invited to attend management planning meetings.

B.3 At the hospital

The emphasis of media attention will often shift from the scene to the hospitals after the initial rescue phase. The hospital's management should activate the hospital's media centre where the media can assemble, obtain refreshment and be briefed at regular intervals. Telephones should be available (direct line, avoiding the hospital switchboard). As at the scene, considerate timing of briefings 30–60 minutes before the main news bulletins will be appreciated and will encourage cooperation.

Senior medical and nursing staff should be aware of the vulnerability of patients, relatives and staff to intrusive interviews and should not allow such interviews to interfere with the welfare of patients and the delivery of care. Statements relating to the condition of individual patients or the hospital's response to the major incident are best made by a nominated hospital spokesperson.

It is also important to monitor individual patient's interactions with the media. Media outlets will contact them through mobile phones and social media. Hospital media teams may be able to offer them and their families advice and support to manage this.

APPENDIX C
Logs

C.1 Introduction

In most domains, the emergency services have a statutory responsibility to respond to and manage major incidents. This will be subject to scrutiny after the event and incident commanders at all levels must be in a position to provide evidence that these responsibilities have been discharged.

Organisations have a corporate responsibility to ensure adequate training and exercising has taken place to support this process.

At an inquiry, individuals and their employing organisation will be asked:

- What was your role?
- Were you appropriately trained to undertake this?
- Were your decisions and actions justifiable?
- Do your logs confirm this?

In order to do this, commanders must ensure that contemporaneous records are maintained throughout the incident.

C.2 Record keeping

Good record keeping does not happen by accident and commanders must be appropriately trained in it.

Records may take the form shown in Box C.1.

Box C.1 Record keeping

- Written/policy logs
- Contemporaneous notes
- Control room logs
- Voice recordings on and off site
- Electronic logs
- Video evidence

The logs must include the times at which events occurred, what was decided and why, who was consulted and at what level, how decisions were implemented and whether decisions were reviewed, and whether checks on implementation occurred.

The rationale for decisions is likely to be evaluated. In particular, evidence of review and evaluation, options appraisal, consultation with others, consideration of outcomes and assurances about effectiveness of implementation will be challenged.

Major Incident Medical Management and Support: The Practical Approach at the Scene, Fourth Edition.
Edited by Tony Gleeson and Kevin Mackway-Jones.
© 2023 John Wiley & Sons Ltd. Published 2023 by John Wiley & Sons Ltd.

Written/policy logs

Written logs are the most common form of record keeping by commanders. Most emergency services carry pre-printed logbooks as part of their response equipment.

Inquiries have often commented on the inadequacy of record keeping.

> 'Unfortunately, it is not possible to examine in detail the London Ambulance Service's response to the Edgware Road explosion . . . because **records of the response were not maintained**. The time line **provided to us** by the London Ambulance Service contains **no entries** beyond 9.21 am . . . This failure to maintain records is not unique to the Ambulance Service; the London Fire Brigade has also commented . . . on the failure to record information about its response and the need to do so in future.' [emphasis added]
>
> *London Assembly Report of the 7 July Review Committee, 6 June 2006*

As part of their planning, organisations need to ensure facilities exist to undertake this logging function. This may require commanders to have a dedicated 'Loggist' from early in the incident.

The role of the Loggist is a critical function to which specialist training is a requirement.

Contemporaneous notes

Where dedicated trained loggists are not available commanders may be required to note their individual logs in a notebook.

In this case the commander must ensure:

- The entry must be:
  - **C**lear
  - **I**ntelligible
  - **A**ccurate
- Each entry in the log should be identified by a sequential reference number
- A record of the date and time of the entry should be made using the 24-hour clock
- All entries should be made in permanent black ink
- No erasures should be made:
  - Mistakes must be ruled through with a single line and initialed
  - No overwriting or writing above the ruled error must be made
  - Correction fluid must not be used in any circumstances

The submission of the incident log following the individual's response to the incident will usually be 48–72 hours post completion of the incident response.

Control room logs

In many countries, voice recordings (from initial calls to the end of the incident) will be made automatically. Additional logs, including command and control for a major incident, may also be undertaken by control room staff.

Incident commanders may establish additional control room logs to record further information regarding the incident.

Voice recordings on and off site

Voice records may be used outside the control room environment using portable recorders. The likely quality of these recording should be considered. These should not be used as the primary logging system.

Electronic logs

Depending on resources available there may be an opportunity to have scribes detailing log entries electronically. Robust back-up systems are required and data protection issues must be considered.

Video evidence

Video information may be recorded by the emergency services, media or the public and provided as evidence after the event.

Key point

Information recorded after the event will not have the same weight as records made at the time.

C.3 After the event

Immediate

As soon as practically possible, copies of any logs should be made by each organisation as the original logs may be required as evidence.

Later

Major incidents will often be the subject of some form of formal inquiry. Commanders will be accountable at several levels, for example:

- Internal major incident review
- Public inquiry
- Coroner's inquest
- Parliamentary inquiry
- Criminal prosecution
- Media scrutiny

These are often high-pressure events; however, the better the quality of recording of the history of events, the less stressful this is likely to be. Actions will be judged on the rationality and reasonableness of the decisions, and this will often be established in light of the evidence from the logs. It is likely that the formal inquiry will occur many months or even years after the event and the reliance on good contemporaneous notes will become more important than ever, as memories of the event will have changed over time.

APPENDIX D
Radio use and voice procedures

D.1 Introduction

The responsibility of the issue of radios for medical responders at a major incident normally lies with the ambulance service. It is essential that communications are structured and controlled by the emergency services and for that reason the use of personal devices are discouraged.

After reading this appendix you should understand the techniques used to carry out the following practical procedures (section D.2) and voice procedure (section D.3).

This appendix will discuss the use of very high frequency (VHF) radios, ultra high frequency (UHF) radios and digital hand-held terminals. The process of voice procedure does not differ but the practical procedures will (see Chapter 13).

D.2 Practical procedures

Box D.1 Practical procedures

- Turning the radio on and transmitting a message
- Changing the radio battery

Turning the radio on and transmitting a message

The reader should refer to Figure D.1, which shows a hand portable VHF radio. However, it is important that users become familiar with the design and function of the types of radios used in their area.

1. Turn the radio on; many models will produce an audible 'beep'.
2. Select the channel/talkgroup you require.

Local highlights: Channel usage

Major Incident Medical Management and Support: The Practical Approach at the Scene, Fourth Edition.
Edited by Tony Gleeson and Kevin Mackway-Jones.
© 2023 John Wiley & Sons Ltd. Published 2023 by John Wiley & Sons Ltd.

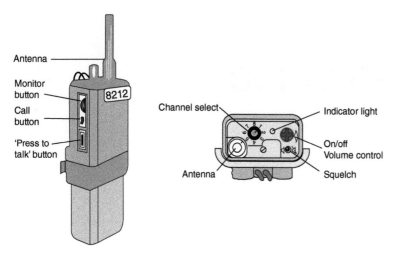

Figure D.1 The VHF radio working parts

3. *Listen* (or *look* at the 'channel busy' light) before transmitting to ensure that the channel is clear.
4. Transmit by depressing the 'press to talk' (PTT) button on the side of radio. Wait 1 second before starting the message.
5. Hold the radio upright about 4–5 cm from your mouth and speak.
6. Release the PTT button to listen to the reply.

Changing the radio battery

If the messages you receive are crackled or broken, it is likely that the battery is low. Some radios will show a 'battery low' warning on the display screen and/or give an audible warning. If the battery is low, change it as follows:

1. Turn the radio off.
2. Engage the battery release switch and remove the battery.
3. Replace with a new battery.
4. Turn on the radio.
5. Perform a radio check.

D.3 Voice procedure

Box D.2 Voice procedure

- **Principles**
- **Radio shorthand**
  - Glossary
  - Phonetic alphabet
  - Numbers and figures
- **Basic message handling**
  - Initiating a call
  - Replying to a call
  - Replying to a group call
  - Ending a message
  - Offering a message
- **Advanced message handling**
  - Corrections
  - Repeating a message
  - Long messages
  - Relaying a message
- **The radio check**

Principles

The fundamentals of a good radio message are:

- **C**larity
- **A**ccuracy
- **B**revity

Clarity can be achieved by attention to the following characteristics of the voice:

- **R**hythm
- **S**peed
- **V**olume
- **P**itch

Remember RSVP.

The *rhythm* should be steady; the *speed* should be slightly slower than normal speech; for adequate *volume* it is not necessary to shout but whispering will be ineffective unless the radio has a specific whisper mode; and the best *pitch* is that of a female voice, so men (with lower voices) should make a conscious effort to raise their pitch.

To achieve *accuracy* and *brevity* requires discipline and practice. Air time is a valuable commodity. The system of radio voice procedure shown in this book is based on military voice procedure but examples of alternative systems are given where appropriate.

Radio shorthand

Glossary

Brevity can be facilitated by using a number of special words that act as a verbal shorthand. These are given in Box D.3.

Box D.3 Radio shorthand	
Over	The speaker now wishes the receiver to talk
Out	The conversation is finished
OK	I understand
Roger	I understand
Yes Yes	Message confirmed
Go ahead	I am ready to receive your message
Send	I am ready to receive your message
Acknowledge	Tell me you have received my message
Say again	Repeat what you said
ETA	Estimated time of arrival
ETD	Estimated time of departure
Wait	I cannot reply within the next five seconds
Wait out	I cannot reply, I will contact you later
Standby	Stay alert, further information to follow

Other words may be in use locally. If so, it is essential that their full meaning is known and understood by all the users of the net.

Local highlights: Local radio shorthand phrases or words

The following terminology is *not* acceptable (Box D.4).

Box D.4 Unacceptable radio shorthand

Over and out	It is either over or out
Rodger dodger	Slang
Ten four	Slang

It is also not appropriate to swear on the radio and it is advisable to avoid comedy ('send the Rover over, over!'). It is wise to remember that the radio net will be monitored by Ambulance Control and messages will be recorded and will be analysed in any subsequent inquiry.

Phonetic alphabet

Difficult or important words should be spelt to avoid confusion. Rather than saying 'ay, bee, see, dee' a phonetic alphabet is used to give each letter a distinct sound: 'alpha, bravo, charlie, delta . . .'. These are listed in Box D.5.

Box D.5 The International Radiotelephony Spelling Alphabet, commonly known as the NATO phonetic alphabet

A	Alpha	**N**	November
B	Bravo	**O**	Oscar
C	Charlie	**P**	Papa
D	Delta	**Q**	Quebec
E	Echo	**R**	Romeo
F	Foxtrot	**S**	Sierra
G	Golf	**T**	Tango
H	Hotel	**U**	Uniform
I	India	**V**	Victor
J	Juliet	**W**	Whiskey
K	Kilo	**X**	X-ray
L	Lima	**Y**	Yankee
M	Mike	**Z**	Zulu

Numbers

For accuracy, the pronunciation of numbers is stressed (Box D.6). Long numbers are spoken whole, then repeated digit by digit.

Box D.6 Number pronunciation

1	Wun	**6**	Six
2	Too	**7**	Seven
3	Thuree	**8**	Ate
4	Fower	**9**	Niner
5	Fiyiv	**0**	Zero

It should be stressed that although this is the ideal method of pronouncing numbers, it can be as easily achieved by saying each number clearly and with limited accent.

A common mistake is to add an 'a' to the end of each number, for example wuna, tooa, thureea, etc. and this should be avoided.

Key example

Mike One, I have nineteen, figures wun-niner, casualties for evacuation, over.
Control, Roger, figures wun-niner casualties for evacuation, over.
Mike One, OK, over.
Control, out.

Basic message handling

Initiating a call

1. To start a message, say the call-sign of the recipient being called (this would normally be a control function.
2. Next state who you are.
3. Finish the message with 'over' (to indicate that the other station can now speak).

Key example

Control, from Mike One, over.

It is also acceptable to initiate a message in the following ways:

- Mike One to Control, over.
- Hello Control, this is Mike One, over.

Replying to a call

Prefix each message you send with your own call-sign.

Key example

Control, go ahead, over.
Mike One, send resupply of bandages to Casualty Clearing Station, over.

Replying to a group call

Occasionally Control or another station will call all the stations on the net. Replies should be in alpha-numerical order. Each station is allowed 5 seconds during which to reply. After this time the next station should reply.

Key example

All stations Mike from Control, acknowledge my last message, over.
Mike One, OK, over.
Mike Two, OK, over.
5-second pause
Mike Four, OK, over.
Control, OK, out to you Mikes One, Two and Four, Mike Three from Control, acknowledge my last message, over.
Mike Three, OK, over.
Control, OK, out.

Note the use of the phrase 'out to you' in this example to indicate to selected stations that there is no further requirement to reply.

Ending a message

A conversation can be finished by using the word 'out'. Only one user needs to say 'out'.

With twin frequency transmissions it is important that Ambulance Control always says 'out', even where Control did not initiate the message. This is because all stations can hear Control but not each other and will wait until they hear the word 'out' to know that they can send a message. This becomes unnecessary when transmitting on an open channel but it is still appropriate to maintain radio discipline.

> **Key example**
>
> Mike One, end of message, over.
> Control, Roger, out.

Offering a message

Theoretically, on a constantly monitored radio net it should not be necessary to 'offer' a message. That is to say, you should be able to move straight into the text of the message. However, experience shows that messages *do* need to be offered as the recipient is not always fully alert and may not be in a position to write things down.

1. Initiate the call as shown above.
2. Indicate that you have a message to send.
3. Finish the transmission with 'over'.
4. Send your message when prompted.

> **Key example**
>
> Control from Mike One, message, over.
> Control, go ahead, over.
> Mike One, require resupply of dressings at Casualty Clearing Station, over.
> Control, Roger, resupply in figures one-zero minutes, over.
> Mike One, OK, out.

Advanced message handling

Corrections

From time to time you will make errors when sending a message. These errors must be corrected as follows:

1. As soon as an error has been made, say 'wrong'.
2. Follow this with the correct message.
3. If necessary, repeat the correct message for clarity.

> **Key example**
>
> Control from Mike One, I have now moved to grid figures three-two-one-seven-six, **wrong**, grid three-two-one-***two***-seven-six, **I say again** three-two-one-two-seven-six, over.
> Control, three-two-one-two-seven-six, over.
> Mike One, correct, out.

Repeating a message

On a military radio net the instruction 'say again' is used for a message to be repeated; 'repeat' is reserved for artillery to fire again! On a civilian net it is acceptable to say 'repeat' to have a message repeated.

1. As soon as the message ends (and the sender says 'over') ask for the message to be repeated.
2. Finish your transmission with 'over' and wait for the repeat.

Key example

Mike One from Control, move now to command vehicle, over.
Mike One, say again, over.
Control, move now to command vehicle, over.
Mike One, Roger, over.
Control, out.

Repeating messages wastes air time. It is critical that individuals monitor their radio constantly so that message are picked up on their first transmission. If only part of a message needs to be repeated, the part that requires repeating should be specified (Box D.7).

Box D.7 Instructions for repeating part of a message

Say again all after   Repeat everything after the specified word
Say again all before   Repeat everything before the specified word
Say again all between   Repeat everything between the specified words

---

Key example

Mike One from Control, incident commanders briefing at police command vehicle in figures two-zero minutes, over.
Mike One, say again all after **police**, over.
Control, command vehicle in figures two-zero minutes, over.
Mike One, Roger, over.
Control, out.

Long messages

Occasionally it is necessary to send a long message on the radio. A METHANE message is an example of this (see Chapter 14). Long messages should be broken down into a series of shorter messages and the receiver should be asked to acknowledge that they have received each part. Not only does this ensure accuracy but it gives the opportunity for others on the net to interrupt if they have a more urgent message.

Some emergency service radios are programmed to break transmission after a fixed time (for example 20–30 seconds), although this is unusual for ambulance service radios.

1. Offer a message and indicate that a 'long message' is to follow.
2. At frequent intervals (never longer than 30 seconds) ask the receiving station to 'acknowledge so far'.
3. Repeat any message fragment not received.
4. When certain that the message fragment has been correctly received, send the next part of the message.
5. Repeat steps 2 to 4 until the entire message has been sent.
6. End the message.

Key example

Control from Mike One, long message, over.

Control, go ahead, over.

Mike One, major incident declared time and figures one-five-zero-zero hours, over. Control, major incident declared, over.

Mike One, exact location, railway cutting two miles west of Farnham, grid figures two-six-five-six-nine, over.

Control, exact location, railway cutting two miles west of Farnham, grid figures two-six-five-six-nine, over.

Mike One, passenger train derailment, fire present and potential electricity hazard, over.

Control, you have passenger train derailment, with fire and potential electricity hazard, over.

Mike One, access via Lord Road, spell Lima-Oscar-Romeo-Delta, Road from the south, rendezvous at Queen Victoria Public House, over.

Control, access via Lord Road from the south, rendezvous at Queen Victoria Public House, over.

Mike One, number of casualties estimated figures two-zero-zero, all services required, make ambulances twenty, over.

Control, number of casualties estimated figures two-zero-zero, all services required, make ambulances twenty, over.

Mike One, message ends, standby for further information, out.

Relaying a message

If all call-signs are not in contact with Control, it is sometimes necessary for messages to be passed to one call-sign via another. Each stage of this process must be accurate.

1. The initiator of the message offers a message to an intermediary.
2. The initiator indicates that message is to be passed to another call-sign (the final recipient).
3. The message is passed to the intermediary.
4. The intermediary acknowledges the messages and ends the call with the initiator.
5. The intermediary offers the message to the final recipient and indicates that the message is being passed from the initiator.
6. The message is passed to the final recipient.
7. The intermediary ends the call to the final recipient.
8. The intermediary calls the initiator and indicates that the message has been passed.

Key example

Mike One from Control, message for Mike Four, over.

Mike One, send, over.

Control, message for Mike Four, send two drug packs to the first carriage, over.

Mike One, OK, out to you . . . Mike Four from Mike One, message from Control, over. Mike Four, send, over.

Mike One, from Control, send two drug packs to the first carriage, over.

Mike Four, OK, over.

Mike One, out to you . . . Control from Mike One, message passed, over.

Control, Roger, out.

The radio check and signal strength

It is important that all call-signs on a net know that they can communicate reliably with Control. This is achieved using the *radio check*. Radio checks can be initiated by Control or by other call-signs.

1. Initiate a call to the station or group of stations to be checked.
2. Indicate that a 'radio check' is being performed.
3. Finish the message with 'over'.
4. Await replies.
5. Indicate the results of the check to the station group of stations.
6. End the call.

Key example

All stations Mike from Control, radio check, over.
Mike One, OK, over.
Mike Two, OK, over.
Mike Three, OK, over.
Control, OK, out.

Stations should answer in numerical sequence with up to 5 seconds between stations (at 5 seconds the next station in sequence should answer). If a station cannot be clearly heard, the key words in Box D.8 are used.

Box D.8 Key words when the radio check is not OK

Difficult	Most words are heard but there is interference
Broken	Messages are heard intermittently
Unworkable	Only occasional words are heard – or interference only
Nothing heard	Nothing is heard at all

APPENDIX E
The hospital response

E.1 Introduction

Major Incident Medical Management and Support: the practical approach in the hospital, outlines for readers the hospital's response to a major incident, while this appendix provides an introduction for pre-hospital providers. The fundamental principles of CSCATTT apply in the hospital setting as they do in the pre-hospital environment. The hospital response can be divided into four phases – preparation, reception, definitive care and recovery:

Preparation involves preparing the hospital to receive casualties from the scene (and will involve the development of the major incident plan well before the incident occurs).

Reception is the receipt of casualties from the scene. Patients may arrive from the scene by their own means or by ambulance. The initial receiving area is the Emergency Department although the theatres, receiving wards and intensive care units will need to be prepared to receive casualties.

Definitive care is the care of patients in the weeks and months post incident.

Recovery is the process of recovering from the incident response and returning to normal care of patients. It involves a review and audit of the incident response.

E.2 Command and control

All hospital plans should specify the individuals who are in control of the response, including how early the on-site controllers will hand over control to senior personnel. The response will be coordinated by a hospital coordination team consisting of a senior doctor, a senior nurse and a senior manager, each of which will be responsible for their own area – medical, nursing and management respectively. A senior Emergency Department (ED) Consultant will also be a part of the hospital coordination team especially in the reception phase of the incident.

Local highlights: Command and control of the hospital response

---

Key point

The health service response at the hospital is controlled by the hospital coordination team.

Major Incident Medical Management and Support: The Practical Approach at the Scene, Fourth Edition.
Edited by Tony Gleeson and Kevin Mackway-Jones.
© 2023 John Wiley & Sons Ltd. Published 2023 by John Wiley & Sons Ltd.

E.3 Key areas

A senior nurse should ensure that the clinical areas (Box E.1) are prepared to receive casualties and should delegate the running of each area to a senior nurse in that area which creates a vertical method of reporting, similar to the vertical reporting seen in each of the services in the pre-hospital environment. Similar vertical command processes are put in place with the medical and management areas of the hospital response.

Box E.1 Key clinical areas

- Triage
- Priority 1 (**immediate**) and 2 (**urgent**)
- Priority 3 (**delayed**)
- Pre-operative and post-operative ward
- Admissions ward
- Theatres
- Intensive care

A senior manager will be responsible for coordinating the non-clinical areas and requirements:

- Activation of staff call in process
- Staff and volunteer reporting area
- Hospital information centre
- Discharge and reunion area: relatives/friends of those getting discharged can wait here
- Bereaved relatives area: counselling
- Press area for media briefings
- Blood donation: if required

E.4 Staff call-in

Each incident response plan will outline the process for the staff call-in system for their department. Staff will be called in using a cascade system that will be activated through switchboard by the senior manager. Staff will be called based on role rather than name, and those key staff called first will arrange for others from their department to be called. The switchboard call-in list will typically represent those on call and those senior individuals from medicine, nursing and management. It then becomes their responsibility to ensure further call-in of individuals from their speciality/area of expertise. This may be delegated. Where possible, this should be done via direct line, mobile phone or even by staff calling each other from home in order to avoid overloading an already stretched switchboard. Staff lists should be regularly assessed and updated. Previously established group messages may also be distributed to avoid hospital lines.

E.5 Preparation

Areas identified for immediate reception of casualties should be cleared as far as is possible. A senior ED clinician should assess all patients in the Emergency Department and decide whether they need admission or whether they can be safely discharged to an alternative source of appropriate care, such as their General Practitioner, or an out-patients clinic in the following days. Patients needing admission need to be moved to an appropriate area in the hospital where they can be assessed further by in-patient teams.

Pre- and post-operative wards will also need to be cleared to gain capacity, and inpatients currently in these designated wards should be discharged where appropriate or moved to a low dependency area. This can be achieved by ensuring ward rounds take place by senior clinicians in each speciality, not only in the receiving wards but in all wards within the hospital.

E.6 Action cards

On arriving at the hospital, staff should attend the staff reporting points for task allocation. Staff roles and responsibilities will be outlined comprehensively in the disaster plan; action cards (Figure E.1) also need to be accessible to all responding staff. These should give a reminder of each person's key responsibilities and a brief description of the duties that they need to perform.

ACTION CARD SENIOR EMERGENCY PHYSICIAN

Responsibilities

- Overall control of the reception areas
- Staffing of key appointments in the reception areas
- Control of initial reception and management
- Initial triage of major incident casualties
- Assistance to the Medical Coordinator after the reception phase has ended
- Operational debriefing of emergency department medical staff involved in the major incident response

Immediate action

- Assume control of the reception areas   Completed by: Time
- Ensure preparation of the reception areas is complete   Completed by: Time
- Ensure that the following posts are filled: senior surgeon and senior physician
  If not appoint a suitably senior doctor until the key personnel arrive   Completed by: Time
- Assess the number of casualty treatment teams required immediately in the reception areas and
  inform the Medical Coordinator   Completed by: Time
- Ensure major incident casualties are triaged as follows:

  Priority 1, immediate: casualties requiring immediate life-saving procedures
  Priority 2, urgent: casualties who will require surgery or other intervention within 6 hours
  Priority 3, delayed: less serious cases not requiring immediate treatment   Completed by: Time

- Continue to assess the situation and, if necessary, establish a further priority as follows:

  Priority 4, expectant: casualties whose injuries are so severe that they cannot survive in the
  circumstances   Completed by: Time

- As further casualty treatment teams are required inform the Medical Coordinator   Completed by: Time
- As casualty transfer teams are required inform the Medical Coordinator   Completed by: Time
- Liaise with the senior nurse in the emergency department regarding senior nurse staffing
  and supplies in the reception areas   Completed by: Time
- Liaise with the Senior Duty Clerk in the emergency department regarding documentation in
  the reception areas   Completed by: Time
- Constantly monitor the triage, treatment, staffing, documentation and supplies in the reception
  areas   Completed by: Time
- Once the reception phase is over assist the Medical Coordinator to control the hospital response   Completed by: Time

Priorities during the incident

- Overall control of the reception areas
- Triage in the reception areas
- Control of staffing in the reception areas
- Control of treatment in the reception areas
- Control of documentation in the reception areas
- Control of supplies in the reception areas
- Assisting the Medical Coordinator to control the hospital response

---

Figure E.1 Example of an action card for a senior emergency physician

E.7 Team organisation

The effective management of the hospital response is centered on the organisation of personnel into teams with specific tasks. These teams include the following:

- Casualty treatment teams
- Casualty transfer teams
- Operating teams

A team coordinator will be based in the reporting area and will have command over the treatment and transfer teams. They will form medical and nursing staff into teams as they become available.

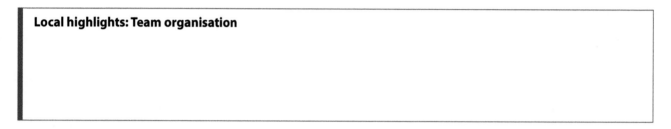

Local highlights: Team organisation

Key point

An effective hospital response is centred around forming personnel into teams with particular tasks.

E.8 Treatment

The nature of the major incident will determine the type of injuries that will present to the hospital. During all major incidents there will be requirement for both surgical and medical capacity. Team composition will have to reflect the nature of the demand.

Clinical activity in each area will be controlled by senior clinicians.

Priority groups

Patients are re-triaged as they arrive in to the hospital and are sent to an appropriate receiving area. In the same way that casualties in the Casualty Clearing Station are divided into priority 1, priority 2 and priority 3, patients arriving will be sent to the P1, P2 and P3 areas in the hospital. Generally, P1 patients will be sent to the Resus room of the department, P2 to other areas in the department and P3 to the minors area of the department or an adjacent out-patients area. Each of these areas will have a lead doctor and nurse who will report to the overall lead doctor/nurse in the ED. A senior surgeon and a senior physician – (usually the duty consultant surgeon and either ICU or duty physician) will be available to support the ED lead for each of the areas in directing the treatment and transfer teams.

Surgical

- The senior surgeon should ensure that the highest priority surgical casualties are transferred directly to the operating theatres
- Once the capacity of the theatres is reached then further casualties should wait for surgery on the pre-operative ward
- The senior surgeon should also appoint deputies to oversee activity in the operating theatres and on the pre-operative ward
- The senior surgeon in theatres will coordinate the operating teams, and any specialist surgeons needed for particular procedures
- The senior surgeon in pre-op will coordinate the treatment teams on the pre-operative ward
- The senior nurse should ensure that all areas are adequately prepared and stocked, and that staffing is adequate

Both will keep the senior surgeon informed of surgical matters in their area.

Medical

- The senior physician should direct the transfer of the most seriously ill patients to the intensive care unit
- The duty intensive care consultant should assess the bed availability in the department and in surrounding hospitals; and organise transfer of patients to other departments

Those casualties who do not require immediate surgery or intensive care facilities will be transferred to an admissions ward.

> **Local highlights: Hospital treatment**

E.9 Staff responsibilities

Emergency department

If a major incident has not been identified by the ambulance service, or if casualties begin to rapidly self-present to hospital, then it is the responsibility of the emergency department to activate and declare a major incident. In some instances, it may be necessary only to activate a limited response of additional emergency department staff – this would be performed by the duty emergency physician.

Medical and nursing staff who are assigned to work in the treatment and transfer teams based in the emergency department will be unfamiliar with this area. To reduce confusion, regular emergency department staff should be visually accessible by wearing tabards in order to provide assistance to such colleagues.

Other departments

A communication cascade system should be used in the event of a disaster to call in staff from home or other areas in the hospital. A staff member may be nominated to call in those who are off duty, again making efforts to minimise the load on the hospital switchboard.

On arrival at the hospital, staff should present to the staff reporting area rather than their usual place of work, since they may be directed to another area that is different to their usual ward. These staff will be logged, given their action cards and allocated roles and responsibilities by the Team Coordinator.

Transfer teams are required to look after priority 1 and 2 patients during transfer from the high dependency areas to the operating rooms, pre-operative ward or intensive care unit. Additionally, teams might be utilised for secondary interhospital transfers.

E.10 Documentation

At the scene the casualty will have a triage label attached to them. Depending on the available resources, clinical information may also be attached to casualties at the scene. This documentation needs to remain with the patient as it will have important information regarding the clinical details, injuries and treatment.

In the initial reception area, each patient will be issued with major incident documentation and given an identification band with the corresponding number, which must not be removed under any circumstances. The senior nurse in each of the treatment areas is responsible for completing a casualty statement form at regular intervals and returning this to the Hospital Information Centre, the Admissions Officer can then maintain an accurate casualty state board.

APPENDIX F
Human factors

F.1 Introduction

The emphasis on major incident medical management has traditionally concentrated on knowledge of the casualty management process, for example, the triage priority being assigned. An often overlooked element is how, in these high-pressure situations, individuals from a variety of different professional and specialty backgrounds come together to form an effective team that minimises errors and works actively to prevent adverse events.

This appendix provides a brief introduction to some of the human factors that can affect the performance of individuals and teams in the healthcare environment. Human factors, also referred to as ergonomics, is an established scientific discipline and clinical human factors has been described as:

Enhancing clinical performance through an understanding of the effects of teamwork, tasks, equipment, workspace, culture and organisation on human behaviour and abilities and application of that knowledge in clinical settings.

(Kohn et al., 2010)

F.2 Extent of healthcare error

In 2000, an influential report entitled *To Err is Human: Building a Safer Health System* (Kohn et al., 2010) suggested that across the USA somewhere between 44 000 and 98 000 deaths each year could be attributed to medical error. A pilot study in the UK demonstrated that approximately one in 10 patients admitted to healthcare experienced an adverse event.

Healthcare has been able to learn from a number of other high-risk industries including the nuclear, petrochemical, space exploration, military and aviation industries about how team issues have been managed. These lessons have been slowly adopted and translated to healthcare.

Specialist working groups and national bodies have been instrumental in promoting awareness of the importance of human factors in healthcare. They aim to raise awareness and promote the principles and practices of human factors; identify current human factor activity, capability and barriers; and create conditions to support human factors being embedded at a local level. One such example of this in the UK is the Human Factors Clinical Working Group and the National Quality Board's concordat statement on human factors.

> **Local highlights: Specialist groups/national bodies promoting awareness of human factors in healthcare**

Major Incident Medical Management and Support: The Practical Approach at the Scene, Fourth Edition.
Edited by Tony Gleeson and Kevin Mackway-Jones.
© 2023 John Wiley & Sons Ltd. Published 2023 by John Wiley & Sons Ltd.

F.3 Causes of healthcare error

Humans make mistakes. No amount of checks and procedures will mitigate this fact. In fact, the only way to completely remove human error is to remove all the humans involved. It is vital therefore to look to work in a way that, wherever possible, minimises the occurrence of mistakes and ensures that when they do occur the method minimises the chance of the error resulting in an adverse event.

F.4 Error chains

Casualty safety errors do not usually occur because of single mistakes. Behind any identified error (A) that leads to an untoward event (B), there is a sequence of factors that set up the conditions such that error A resulted in event B and without which event B would not have occurred.

It has been suggested that these human errors can be further categorised into:

1. Those that occur at the sharp end of care by the treating team and individuals.
2. Those that occur at the blunt or organisational level, typically through policies and procedures.

It is typically found that the latent/organisational issues often coexist with the sharp errors; in fact, it is rare for an isolated error to occur – often there is a chain of events that results in the adverse event. The 'Swiss cheese' model demonstrates how apparently random, unconnected events and organisational decisions can all make errors more likely (Figure F.1). Conversely, a standardised system with good defences can capture these errors and prevent adverse events.

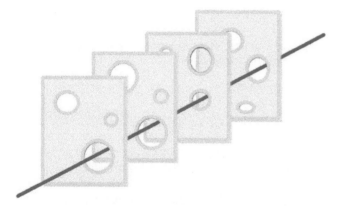

Figure F.1 The 'Swiss cheese' model

Each of the slices of Swiss cheese represents barriers that, under ideal circumstances, would prevent or detect the error. The holes represent weaknesses in these barriers: if the holes align the error passes through undetected.

The end result is that multiple defences have been weakened or removed, and the error is more likely to cause harm. It is also important to be aware of the different types of error: potential gaps in knowledge, a latent/organisational error (no effective policy and possibly an issue with staffing) and a routine violation.

F.5 Learning from error

Historically, those making mistakes have been identified and singled out for punishment and/or retraining, in what is often referred to as a culture of blame. Does retraining these individuals make it safer for other or future casualties? That clearly depends on the underlying reasons. If it was purely a knowledge gap, possibly, but does the same knowledge gap exist elsewhere? Potentially all the other issues remain unresolved. Moreover, such punitive reactions make it less likely for individuals to admit mistakes and near misses in the future.

The focus is now on learning from error and, in shifting away from the individual, is much more focused on determining the system/organisational errors. Once robust systems, procedures and policies that work and are effective are in place, then errors can be captured. Of course, issues will still need to be addressed where individuals have been reckless or lacked knowledge – but now reasons why the individuals felt the need to violate, or had not been given all the knowledge required, can be looked at.

For this to work, health services need to learn from errors, adverse events and near misses. This requires engagement at both the individual level, by reporting errors, and the organisational level, investigating and feeding back the error using a systematic approach. It is also key that information is cascaded through the organisation and across the health service to raise awareness and prevent similar situations.

Violation may be indicative of the failure of systems, procedures or policies or other cultural issues. It is important that policies, procedures, roles and even our buildings and equipment are all designed pro-actively with human factors in mind, so things do not have to be fixed retrospectively when adverse events occur. This means that all members of the organisation must be aware of human factors, not just the front-line emergency staff.

Improving team and individual performance

Having discussed the magnitude of the problem of healthcare error, the rest of this appendix will focus on how the performance of teams and individuals can be developed.

Raising awareness of the human factors, and being able to practise these skills and behaviours within multiprofessional teams, allows the development of effective teams in all situations. Simulation activity allows a team to explore these new ideas, practise them and develop them. To do this we need feedback on our performance within a safe environment where no casualty is at risk and egos and personal interests can be set aside.

Consider how you developed a clinical skill. It was something that needed to be practised again and again until eventually it started to become automatic and routine. The same applies for our human factor behaviours. In addition, recognising our inherent human limitations and the situations when errors are more likely to occur, we can all be hyper-vigilant when required.

F.6 Communication

Poor communication is the leading cause of adverse events. This is not surprising; to have an effective team there needs to be good communication. The leader needs to communicate with the followers, and followers communicate with leaders and other followers. Communication is not just saying something – it is ensuring that information is accurately passed on and received. We all want to ensure effective communication at all times. Remember there are multiple components to effective communication (Table F.1).

Table F.1 Elements of communication				
Sender	**Sender**	**Transmitted**	**Receiver**	**Receiver**
Thinks of what to say	Says message	Through air, over phone, via email	Hears it	Thinks about it and acts

The resulting outcome in a noisy, highly pressured major incident can be poor information exchange.

When communicating face-to-face a lot of the information is transmitted non-verbally, which can make telephone or email conversations more challenging. Communication can be more difficult when talking across professional, speciality or hierarchical barriers as we do not always talk the same technical language, have the same levels of understanding or even have a full awareness of the other person's role.

There are a variety of similar tools to aid communication, like METHANE (Major incident - standby or declared, Exact location, Type of incident, Hazards, Access to scene, Number and severity of casualties, Emergency services present and required). METHANE is designed for major incident communications. It facilitates the sender to plan and organise the message, make it succinct and focused, and provide it in a logical and expected order. It is also an empowerment tool allowing the sender (who may be more junior) to request an action from a more senior individual. While these tools are useful, they tend to be reserved for certain situations, whereas we want to establish effective communication as the routine not the exception. One method to routinely improve communication is to incorporate a feedback loop.

Effective communication with a feedback loop

A technique that can be easily introduced to generate an improvement in communication is the *feedback loop*. The feedback loop is a process within which the receiver repeats the message back to the sender to acknowledge and clarify that it has been correctly deciphered. It is quick and simple, and easy to implement. We now know that the message has been transmitted and received correctly. For this process to work both parties (the sender and receiver) need to understand and expect it – again demonstrating the need for us to practise and train together.

Body language and hierarchy

It is important to be aware of non-verbal signals. Postures that say 'I'm bored', 'I'm tired' or 'I don't value you' can serve to prevent the passing of a key piece of information. The presence of a rigid hierarchy can be particularly dangerous, promoting a culture where junior staff do not feel empowered to speak directly to senior staff. Whilst clarity in command is important in major incidents, this needs to be balanced against the need to communicate freely.

F.7 Team working, leadership and followership

At a basic level a team is a group of individuals with a common cause. Historically, training tends to be individually or in professional silos; the risk here is that a 'team of experts' are made rather than an 'expert team'. In a major incident, teams often form at short notice and often arrive at different times. Much emphasis has previously been given to the role of the leader, but a leader cannot be a team on their own. As much emphasis should be given to developing the other team members: the active followers. A good leader will be able to swap from the role of leader to follower as more senior staff arrive and agree to take over.

The leader

The leader's role is multifaceted and includes directing the team, assigning tasks and assessing performance, motivating and encouraging the team to work together, and planning and organising. All leadership skills and behaviours need to be developed and practised. There are different leadership styles and the leader needs to choose an appropriate style for that situation. Effective communication is key and should be reviewed and reflected upon regularly. Constructive feedback should both be given and sought, in order to facilitate continuously improving performance.

Who is the leader?

It is vitally important to have a clearly identified leader. There can be times when people come and go, or different specialties arrive, creating a situation where it may not be clear who the leader is. In a major incident the various officers will wear tabards to make it clear which role they are undertaking. A scribe will be logging the events and they should record who is leading and any changes to the leader.

Speaking up

A useful communication tool, utilised by the airline industry, is shown in the following box. This structure can be used by any person who is concerned that they have information that might be important to others in the team. The levels *probe, alert, challenge,* and *emergency* are utilised sequentially to express increasing concern. If a disaster is imminent, it is entirely appropriate to use the challenge or even emergency stages without recourse to the initial ones. This approach becomes even more powerful when embedded in working practice as both the speaker and the listener should recognise the level of the communication and act appropriately.

The probing question allows diplomacy and maintenance of the hierarchy while raising a point.

Stage	Level of concern	
P	Probe	*I think you need to know what is happening*
A	Alert	*I think something bad might happen*
C	Challenge	*I know something bad will happen*
E	Emergency	*I will not let it happen*

F.8 Situational awareness

Good situational awareness is achieved when we have sufficient and correct information, have interpreted it correctly and are able to correctly project the outcome of an intervention into the future based on current knowledge. If there we have insufficient or incomplete information, we may draw the wrong conclusions about what is going on.

The way a particular situation is perceived is affected by the information conveyed via our own senses, our past experience, our level of alertness, our current workload and the influence of intercurrent distractions. A common trap is to only see or register the information that fits in with a current mental model. This is known as *confirmation bias*. When this occurs, information that confirms preconceptions or current hypotheses is favoured regardless of whether the information is true.

It is vital that everyone understands the concept of situational awareness and continually questions their own thought processes and those of others around them. It is also vital that the team share their impressions of the current situation. There is good evidence that the situational awareness of a well-functioning team is actually greater than the sum of its individual parts. This may be in part due to the elimination of bad data. Information or comments by others that challenge a current mental picture should be treated as a trigger to consider whether situational awareness is lacking. A discussion of the disparity should uncover the true picture. Problems occur when individuals either ignore or rationalise the errant data to fit into their current picture of the world rather than treat it as a challenge.

Typically, three levels of situation awareness are described:

- **Level 1** – What is going on?
- **Level 2** – So what?
- **Level 3** – Now what?

Even at **Level 1** – the basic level of perception – we are prone to errors because the risk seen is what is expected to be seen rather than what is there.

Within healthcare, distractions become the norm to such an extent that individuals are often not even aware of them. The risk is that mistakes are made, and information is missed. It is important to try to challenge interruptions when doing critical tasks and, when they do occur, to restart the task from the beginning rather than from where it is considered the interruption occurred. Some organisations are looking at specific quiet areas for critical tasks. Whatever the local set up, the key is to develop and maintain everyone's awareness of how distraction greatly increases the chance of error.

Level 2 captures how someone's understanding forms from what has been seen. To minimise Level 2 errors, consideration is needed as to how the human brain works, recognises things and makes decisions and choices. This level of detail is beyond the scope of this introductory appendix, and therefore this section will focus on a part of this – the decision making that leads into Level 3.

On the face of it, the practice of decision making is familiar to everyone. However, to understand the factors that can compromise this process it is important to understand the factors that will influence the decision made. To make a good decision a person needs to assess all aspects of a problem, identify the possible responses to the problem, consider the consequences of each of those responses and then weigh up the advantages and disadvantages in order to draw a conclusion. Having completed this, they then need to communicate their decision to their team.

Good situational awareness is a basic prerequisite of this process. To achieve this, the decision maker must ensure they have all the key information. The whole team should be on the alert for ambiguities or conflicting information. Any inconsistent facts should be treated as a potential marker for faulty situation awareness. They should never be brushed off as unimportant anomalies in the absence of evidence to support such a decision.

In many clinical situations there can be a significant pressure of time. Where this is not the case, no decision-making process should be concluded until the team is satisfied, they have all the information and have considered all the options. Where time is a pressure, a certain amount of pragmatism must be employed. There is plenty of evidence to confirm that practise and experience can mitigate some of the negative effects of abbreviating a decision-making process. Those making decisions under such circumstances need to remain aware of the shortcuts they have taken. They should be ready to receive feedback from their team, particularly if any member of the team has significant concerns about the proposed course of action.

At **Level 3**, having seen and understood, we can now plan forward and communicate this with the team.

Team situation awareness

The individuals in the team may have a differing awareness of the situation depending on their previous experience, speciality, physical position, etc. The team's situation awareness will often be greater than any one individual's, however this can only be exploited if the individual elements are effectively communicated. The leader should actively encourage this.

F.9 Improving team and individual performance

In addition to effective communication, team working, situation awareness, leadership and followership skills, there are a number of other ways that team and individual performance can be further developed and improved.

Awareness of situations when errors are more likely

If we are aware that errors are more likely, we can be more proactive in detecting them. Two common situations that make errors more likely are stress and fatigue. Stress is not only a source of error when we are overworked and overstimulated, but also at the other end of the spectrum: we become inattentive when we are understimulated.

The acronym HALT has been used to describe situations when error is more likely:

H	Hungry
A	Angry
L	Late
T	Tired

IM SAFE has been used as a checklist in the aviation industry, asking whether the individual may be affected by:

I	Illness
M	Medication
S	Stress
A	Alcohol
F	Fatigue
E	Emotion

Ideally, individuals who are potentially compromised need to be supported appropriately, allowed time to recover and the team made aware. How this can be achieved in the middle of a night shift can be problematic.

Cognitive aids: checklists, guidelines and protocols

Cognitive aids such as guidelines are important because the human memory is not infallible. They also confer team understanding through the use of a standardised response. This reduces stress. This is especially true where an uncommon emergency event occurs. The team may be unfamiliar with one another, and each member will be trying to remember what to do, what treatments are required and in what order. A good team leader will use the available cognitive aids as a prompt and the team's members can use it as a resource so that they can plan ahead. Safe practice is promoted through the use of these tools in an emergency rather than relying on memory.

Using all available resources

Team resources include staff, observations, equipment, cognitive aids and the facilities in the local area. The team leader should continually consider the appropriateness of utilising available, un-tasked staff or equipment to optimise the patient's care and prevent a bottleneck in the treatment pathway.

Debriefing

Wherever possible a debriefing should be facilitated, even briefly, following clinical events. Ideally this should be normal procedure, rather than being reserved for catastrophic events. The aim of a debrief is to summarise any particular issues or problems that the team had and reflect on how the team performed. Some organisations have set templates to facilitate this. It gives the opportunity for individuals, teams and organisations to continually develop.

In this appendix a brief introduction to the human factors has been given that can lead to poor team working, patient harm and adverse events. It is really important to use every opportunity to reflect and develop your own performance and influence the development of others and the team.

F.10 References

Bromiley M. *Just a Routine Operation*. https://vimeo.com/970665. Clinical Human Factors Group, www.chfg.co.uk (last accessed July 2022).

Kohn LT, Corrigan JM, Donaldson MS (eds); Institute of Medicine (US) Committee on Quality of Health Care in America. *To Err is Human: Building a Safer Health System*. Washington DC: National Academies Press, 2010.

Template annexe of local highlights

This template annexe of local highlights has been prepared for use in conjunction with *Major Incident Medical Management and Support 4e: the practical approach at the scene.*

The core text has been prepared to provide an internationally recognisable approach to major incident management. In order that the text can be enhanced to contain country- or area-specific information, we have used the concept of 'local highlights' boxes.

A local highlights annexe will be available for each country where the MIMMS course is offered. This will be provided in its local form for course participants and all of the sets of local highlights will be available via the ALSG website www.alsg.org

In some countries there is no national approach to certain aspects of major incident management and where this is the case we have indicated this in the appropriate section. In these instances, you should take the time to investigate the regional or trust approach (as appropriate). You will then be in a position to produce a truly personalised version of the core text.

Major Incident Medical Management and Support: The Practical Approach at the Scene, Fourth Edition.
Edited by Tony Gleeson and Kevin Mackway-Jones.
© 2023 John Wiley & Sons Ltd. Published 2023 by John Wiley & Sons Ltd.

Chapter 1: Introduction

Major incident definitions

Guidance for event planning

Chapter 2: The structured approach to major incidents

Major incident plans

Incident activation

Chapter 3: Health service structure and roles

Title of commanders

Initial report

Ambulance service command structure

Ambulance service key roles

Medical service command structure

Command equipment provision

Mobile medical team capacity and provision

Mobile surgical team capacity and provision

Voluntary aid societies

Chapter 4: Emergency service organisation and roles

Local variance and/or local clarification to MIMMS guidance for this chapter

Chapter 5: Support service organisation and roles

Local variance and/or local clarification to MIMMS guidance for this chapter

Chapter 6: Planning

Local variance and/or local clarification to MIMMS guidance for this chapter

Chapter 7: Personal equipment

Colour schemes for emergency service clothing

Local clothing requirements

Helmet markings and colours

Chapter 8: Medical equipment

Life-saving first aid

Equipment needed for extended paramedic skills

Chapter 9: Training

Local variance and/or local clarification to MIMMS guidance for this chapter

Chapter 10: Command and control

Incident Commander name and identification

Chapter 11: Health service scene layout

Identification of the Health Service Command Point

Equipment for the control of key areas

Chapter 12: Safety at the scene

Relevant health and safety legislation

Chapter 13: Communications

Local variance and/or local clarification to MIMMS guidance for this chapter

Chapter 14: Assessment

Local variance and/or local clarification to MIMMS guidance for this chapter

Chapter 15: Triage

Triage priority

Rules for invoking the expectant category

Paediatric triage

Triage labels in use

Chapter 16: Treatment

Expected qualifications of responders

Chapter 17: Transport

Local variance and/or local clarification to MIMMS guidance for this chapter

Chapter 18: Responsibility for the dead

Local variance and/or local clarification to MIMMS guidance for this chapter

Chapter 19: Hazardous materials and CBRNe incidents

Local variance and/or local clarification to MIMMS guidance for this chapter

Chapter 20: Incidents involving large numbers of children

National guidelines for the needs of children in major incidents

Chapter 21: Incidents involving multiple casualties with burns

Local variance and/or local clarification to MIMMS guidance for this chapter

Chapter 22: Mass gatherings

Mass gatherings – local and national guidelines

Chapter 23: Natural disasters

Local variance and/or local clarification to MIMMS guidance for this chapter

Chapter 24: Uncompensated major incidents

Local variance and/or local clarification to MIMMS guidance for this chapter

Chapter 25: Marauding terrorist attacks

Local variance and/or local clarification to MIMMS guidance for this appendix

Appendix A: Psychological aspects of major incidents

Support and counselling

Appendix B: The media

Local variance and/or local clarification to MIMMS guidance for this appendix

Appendix C: Logs

Local variance and/or local clarification to MIMMS guidance for this appendix

Appendix D: Radio use and voice procedures

Channel usage

Local radio shorthand phrases or words

Appendix E: The hospital response

Command and control of the hospital response

Team organisation

Hospital treatment

Appendix F: Human factors

Specialist groups/national bodies promoting awareness of human factors in healthcare

Glossary

ABC	airway, breathing, circulation
ACP	Ambulance Control Point
AIC	Ambulance Incident Commander
BASICS	British Association for Immediate Care Schemes
BATs	burns advice team
BCM	business continuity management
BSAT	burns specialist advice team
BSCT	burns specialist care team
CBRNe	chemical, biological, radiological, nuclear and explosive
CCO	Casualty Clearing Officer
CCS	Casualty Clearing Station
CPD	continuing professional development
CSCATTT	command, safety, communication, assessment, triage, treatment and transport
ED	Emergency Department
EOD	explosive ordnance disposal
FAC	Forward Ambulance Commander
FC	Fire Commander
FCP	Forward Control Point
FCP	Forward Command Post
FFC	Forward Fire Commander
FIO	Forward Incident Officer
FMC	Forward Medical Commander
FPC	Forward Police Commander
FRS	fire and rescue service
HANE	hazards, access, number of casualties, equipment and staff required
HART	Hazardous Area Response Team
HEMS	Helicopter Emergency Medical Service
HF	high frequency
ICU	Intensive Care Unit

Major Incident Medical Management and Support: The Practical Approach at the Scene, Fourth Edition.
Edited by Tony Gleeson and Kevin Mackway-Jones.
© 2023 John Wiley & Sons Ltd. Published 2023 by John Wiley & Sons Ltd.

IED	improvised explosive devices
JDM	Joint Decision Model
JESCC	Joint Emergency Services Control Centre
JESIP	Joint Emergency Service Interoperability Programme
LMA	laryngeal mask airway
LTOWB	low-titre O whole blood
MA	Medical Advisor
MERITs	Medical Emergency Response Incident Teams
METHANE	major incident, exact location, type of incident, hazards, access/egress, number of casualties and emergency services
MIMMS	*Major Incident Medical Management and Support*
MIO	Medical Incident Officer
MMS	multimedia messaging service
MTA	marauding terrorist attack
MTPAS	Mobile Telephone Preference Access Scheme
NBBBs	National Burns Bed Bureaus
PC	Police Commander
PDA	predetermined attendance
PEWCs	practical exercises without casualties
PPE	personal protective equipment
PTSD	post-traumatic stress disorder
PTT	press to talk
RP	Rendezvous Point
RSVP	rhythm, speed, volume and pitch
SMS	short message service
SORTs	Special Operations Response Teams
TRTS	Triage Revised Trauma Score
UHF	ultra high frequency
USAR	urban search and rescue
VHF	very high frequency

Index

Note: Page references in *italics* refer to figures; those in **bold** refer to tables

Major Incident Medical Management and Support: The Practical Approach at the Scene, Fourth Edition.
Edited by Tony Gleeson and Kevin Mackway-Jones.
© 2023 John Wiley & Sons Ltd. Published 2023 by John Wiley & Sons Ltd.